WESTERN MARYLAND

1. BIG RUN STATE PARK
2. BRUNSWICK FAMILY CAMPGROUND
3. CATOCTIN MOUNTAIN PARK
4. C&O CANAL: DRIVE-IN SITES
5. C&O CANAL: HIKER/BIKER CAMPSITES FROM SWAIN'S LOCK (MILE 16.6) TO KILLIANSBURG CAVE (MILE 75.2)
6. C&O CANAL: HIKER/BIKER CAMPSITES FROM HORSESHOE BEND (MILE 79) TO CACAPON JUNCTION (MILE 133)
7. C&O CANAL: HIKER/BIKER CAMPSITES FROM INDIGO NECK (MILE 139) TO EVITTS CREEK (MILE 180)
8. CUNNINGHAM FALLS STATE PARK: WILLIAM HOUCK AREA
9. CUNNINGHAM FALLS STATE PARK: MANOR AREA
10. DEEP CREEK LAKE STATE PARK: MEADOW MOUNTAIN CAMPGROUND
11. FORT FREDERICK STATE PARK
12. GAMBRILL STATE PARK: ROCK RUN AREA
13. GARRETT STATE FOREST: SNAGGY MOUNTAIN AREA
14. GARRETT STATE FOREST: PINEY MOUNTAIN AREA
15. GREEN RIDGE STATE FOREST: NORTH OF I-68
16. GREEN RIDGE STATE FOREST: WEST OF GREEN RIDGE
17. GREEN RIDGE STATE FOREST: EAST OF GREEN RIDGE
18. GREENBRIER STATE PARK
19. MAPLE TREE CAMP
20. NEW GERMANY STATE PARK
21. POTOMAC STATE FOREST: LOSTLAND RUN AREA AND BACKCOUNTRY CAMPING
22. POTOMAC STATE FOREST: LAUREL RUN AND WALLMAN AREAS
23. ROCKY GAP STATE PARK
24. SAVAGE RIVER STATE FOREST: NORTHEAST OF SR RESERVOIR
25. SAVAGE RIVER STATE FOREST: RESERVOIR AND BIG RUN NORTH
26. SOUTH MOUNTAIN STATE PARK: APPALACHIAN TRAIL SHELTERS
27. SOUTH MOUNTAIN STATE PARK: APPALACHIAN TRAIL BACKPACKERS' CAMPGROUNDS
28. SWALLOW FALLS STATE PARK
29. YOUGHIOGHENY RIVER LAKE: MILL RUN CAMPGROUND

CENTRAL MARYLAND

30. LOUISE F. COSCA REGIONAL PARK
31. CEDARVILLE STATE FOREST
32. ELK NECK STATE PARK
33. GREENBELT PARK
34. HART-MILLER ISLAND
35. LITTLE BENNETT REGIONAL PARK
36. PATAPSCO VALLEY STATE PARK: HILTON AREA
37. PATAPSCO VALLEY STATE PARK: HOLLOFIELD AREA
38. PATUXENT RIVER PARK
39. SUSQUEHANNA STATE PARK

SOUTHERN MARYLAND AND EASTERN SHORE

40. ASSATEAGUE ISLAND NATIONAL SEASHORE: BAYSIDE CAMPGROUND
41. ASSATEAGUE ISLAND NATIONAL SEASHORE: OCEANSIDE CAMPGROUND
42. ASSATEAGUE ISLAND NATIONAL SEASHORE: BACKCOUNTRY SITES
43. ASSATEAGUE STATE PARK
44. JANES ISLAND STATE PARK
45. MARTINAK STATE PARK
46. POCOMOKE RIVER STATE PARK: MILBURN LANDING AREA
47. POCOMOKE RIVER STATE PARK: SHAD LANDING AREA
48. POINT LOOKOUT STATE PARK
49. SMALLWOOD STATE PARK
50. TUCKAHOE STATE PARK

Other titles in this series

The Best in Tent Camping: The Carolinas
The Best in Tent Camping: Colorado
The Best in Tent Camping: Florida
The Best in Tent Camping: Georgia
The Best in Tent Camping: Kentucky
The Best in Tent Camping: Minnesota
The Best in Tent Camping: Missouri and the Ozarks
The Best in Tent Camping: Montana
The Best in Tent Camping: New England
The Best in Tent Camping: New Jersey
The Best in Tent Camping: New Mexico
The Best in Tent Camping: New York State
The Best in Tent Camping: Northern California
The Best in Tent Camping: Oregon
The Best in Tent Camping: Pennsylvania
The Best in Tent Camping: The Southern Appalachian and Smoky Mountains
The Best in Tent Camping: Southern California
The Best in Tent Camping: Tennessee
The Best in Tent Camping: Utah
The Best in Tent Camping: Virginia
The Best in Tent Camping: Washington
The Best in Tent Camping: West Virginia
The Best in Tent Camping: Wisconsin

THE BEST IN TENT CAMPING

A GUIDE FOR CAR CAMPERS WHO HATE RVs,
CONCRETE SLABS, AND LOUD PORTABLE STEREOS

MARYLAND

EVAN BALKAN

MENASHA RIDGE PRESS
BIRMINGHAM, ALABAMA

For Woody—who provides good food, and great conversation

♻ Printed on recycled paper

Library of Congress Cataloging-in-Publication Data

Balkan, Evan, 1972—
    The best in tent camping, Maryland : a guide for car campers who hate RVs,
concrete slabs, and loud portable stereos / by Evan Balkan. -- 1st ed.
        p. cm.
Includes bibliographical references and index.
ISBN-13: 978-0-89732-977-4 (alk. paper)
ISBN-10: 0-89732-977-5 (alk. paper)
    1. Campsites, facilities, etc.—Maryland—Directories. 2. Camping—Maryland—
Guidebooks. 3. Maryland—Guidebooks. I. Title.
GV191.42.M3B35 2008
917.5206'842—dc22
                              2007049417

Cover and text design by Ian Szymkowiak, Palace Press International, Inc.
Cover photo by Jerry and Marcy Monkman / Ecophotography.com / Alamy
Cartography by Steve Jones, Jennie Zehmer and Evan Balkan

Menasha Ridge Press
P.O. Box 43673
Birmingham, Alabama 35243
www.menasharidge.com

TABLE OF CONTENTS

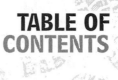

OVERVIEW MAP .... inside front cover
PREFACE vii
ABOUT THE AUTHOR ix
INTRODUCTION 1

WESTERN MARYLAND 9

1. BIG RUN STATE PARK 10
2. BRUNSWICK FAMILY CAMPGROUND 13
3. CATOCTIN MOUNTAIN PARK 16
4. C&O CANAL: DRIVE-IN SITES 19
5. C&O CANAL: HIKER/BIKER CAMPSITES FROM SWAIN'S LOCK (MILE 16.6)
   TO KILLIANSBURG CAVE (MILE 75.2) 23
6. C&O CANAL: HIKER/BIKER CAMPSITES FROM HORSESHOE BEND (MILE 79)
   TO CACAPON JUNCTION (MILE 133) 27
7. C&O CANAL: HIKER/BIKER CAMPSITES FROM INDIGO NECK (MILE 139)
   TO EVITTS CREEK (MILE 180) 30
8. CUNNINGHAM FALLS STATE PARK: WILLIAM HOUCK AREA 33
9. CUNNINGHAM FALLS STATE PARK: MANOR AREA 36
10. DEEP CREEK LAKE STATE PARK: MEADOW MOUNTAIN CAMPGROUND 39
11. FORT FREDERICK STATE PARK 42
12. GAMBRILL STATE PARK: ROCK RUN AREA 45
13. GARRETT STATE FOREST: SNAGGY MOUNTAIN AREA 48
14. GARRETT STATE FOREST: PINEY MOUNTAIN AREA AND BACKCOUNTRY CAMPING ... 51
15. GREEN RIDGE STATE FOREST: NORTH OF I-68 54
16. GREEN RIDGE STATE FOREST: WEST OF GREEN RIDGE 57
17. GREEN RIDGE STATE FOREST: EAST OF GREEN RIDGE 60
18. GREENBRIER STATE PARK 63
19. MAPLE TREE CAMP 66
20. NEW GERMANY STATE PARK 69
21. POTOMAC STATE FOREST: LOSTLAND RUN AREA AND BACKCOUNTRY CAMPING ... 72
22. POTOMAC STATE FOREST: LAUREL RUN AND WALLMAN AREAS 75
23. ROCKY·GAP STATE PARK 78
24. SAVAGE RIVER STATE FOREST: NORTHEAST OF SR RESERVOIR 81
25. SAVAGE RIVER STATE FOREST: RESERVOIR AND BIG RUN NORTH 84
26. SOUTH MOUNTAIN STATE PARK: APPALACHIAN TRAIL SHELTERS 87
27. SOUTH MOUNTAIN STATE PARK: APPALACHIAN TRAIL BACKPACKERS' CAMPGROUNDS ... 91

28. SWALLOW FALLS STATE PARK 94
29. YOUGHIOGHENY RIVER LAKE: MILL RUN CAMPGROUND .97

CENTRAL MARYLAND 101

30. LOUISE F. COSCA REGIONAL PARK 102
31. CEDARVILLE STATE FOREST 105
32. ELK NECK STATE PARK 108
33. GREENBELT PARK 111
34. HART–MILLER ISLAND 114
35. LITTLE BENNETT REGIONAL PARK 117
36. PATAPSCO VALLEY STATE PARK: HILTON AREA 120
37. PATAPSCO VALLEY STATE PARK: HOLLOFIELD AREA 123
38. PATUXENT RIVER PARK 126
39. SUSQUEHANNA STATE PARK 129

SOUTHERN MARYLAND AND EASTERN SHORE 133

40. ASSATEAGUE ISLAND NATIONAL SEASHORE: BAYSIDE CAMPGROUND 134
41. ASSATEAGUE ISLAND NATIONAL SEASHORE: OCEANSIDE CAMPGROUND 137
42. ASSATEAGUE ISLAND NATIONAL SEASHORE: BACKCOUNTRY SITES 140
43. ASSATEAGUE STATE PARK 144
44. JANES ISLAND STATE PARK 146
45. MARTINAK STATE PARK 150
46. POCOMOKE RIVER STATE PARK: MILBURN LANDING AREA 153
47. POCOMOKE RIVER STATE PARK: SHAD LANDING AREA 156
48. POINT LOOKOUT STATE PARK 159
49. SMALLWOOD STATE PARK 162
50. TUCKAHOE STATE PARK 165

APPENDIX AND INDEX 169

CAMPING EQUIPMENT CHECKLIST 171
INDEX 173

PREFACE

I'VE HAD THE GOOD FORTUNE TO TRAVEL quite a bit, visiting some 25 countries on four continents and at least half of the American states. When I travel, comparisons to home are inevitable. Maryland, by most accounts, should come up short. After all, while Maryland enjoys a rich history (I grew up just a mile from a church built in the late 1600s), what is it against Machu Picchu, the Roman Coliseum, or the pyramids at Giza? Maryland's high point tops out at just over 3,300 feet—what's that against major peaks in the Rockies, the Andes, or the Himalayas. Yes, I've spent many happy hours frolicking in the green, pounding surf of the mid-Atlantic off Ocean City, but can it compare to the crystal clarity of Lake Tahoe or the stupendous natural splendor of the Pacific off California's Big Sur?

Believe it or not, I find that invariably, my little Maryland manages to hold its own, thank you very much.

Perhaps an objective judge would find my comparisons ridiculous, and I'll concede that there's something of a hometown bump going on, but I make my favorable judgments without embarrassment. In fact, when I first visited Lake Tahoe and California's Pacific Coast, for example, it was October, and while virtually everything I saw in beautiful northern California was brown and scrubby, I was reminded on my flight home why I love Maryland; during the airplane's descent, I watched with joy as we glided over the spiraling kaleidoscope of color that is autumn in Maryland.

I once read somewhere that when you take into account all of Maryland's tributaries, the state actually has more miles of shoreline than California. I find that claim dubious, though I suppose some favorable formulation will allow you to arrive at that conclusion. Of course, there are so many competing claims for superlatives—for instance, I've seen no fewer than three locales boasting that they are the world's most isolated, populated spots— it seems that the veracity of claims of highest, deepest, wettest, oldest, and so on has to be measured against formulation and whatever particular tourist board is making the assertion. Nevertheless, it is indisputable that if you take the Chesapeake Bay, the Atlantic Ocean, and all the tributaries in the Bay watershed, you could spend a lifetime paddling the shores of all of them. Still, for my money, plunk me down in the mountains and I'm content. Maryland's west is full of great recreational activities, and the camping is no exception.

In short, Marylanders enjoy something of an embarrassment of riches when it comes to the great outdoors. So get out there and enjoy it.

—Evan Balkan

ABOUT THE AUTHOR

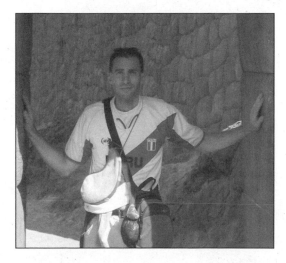

EVAN BALKAN teaches writing at the
Community College of Baltimore County. His
fiction and nonfiction, mostly in the areas of travel
and outdoor recreation, have been published
throughout the United States as well as in Canada,
England, and Australia. A graduate of Towson,
George Mason, and Johns Hopkins universities,
he is also the author of *60 Hikes within 60 Miles:
Baltimore* and *Vanished! Explorers Forever Lost*
(Menasha Ridge Press). He lives in
Lutherville, Maryland, with his wife, Shelly,
and daughters, Amelia and Molly.

MANY MARYLANDERS LIKE TO BOAST about the state's unofficial nickname, "America in Miniature." Bestowed on the state by *National Geographic* founding editor, Gilbert Grosvenor, it's not a hyperbolic moniker. For a relatively small state—the country's ninth smallest in area (with number ten almost twice the size)—Maryland packs in a tremendous amount of diversity. Having both mountains and ocean shoreline in the same state is a real plus for residents; however, many states on the East Coast can make the same claim. What sets Maryland apart from these is the presence of the Chesapeake Bay, the country's largest estuary. The Bay's central and massive presence in Maryland means its effects are far-reaching; in addition to being a major source of recreation, the bay's bounty formed a major part of the state's economy from Maryland's founding in the 17th century all the way through the next three centuries.

Generally, the state is carved by three distinct fault lines, which run geographically as well as politically and culturally: Western Maryland is mountainous and retains some vestiges of its status as part of America's first frontier, the Alleghany range of the Appalachians providing the first natural barrier to European immigrants heading west. Central Maryland is urban and suburban, anchored by Baltimore in the north and Washington, D.C., in the south. The corridor between is home to high-end service industries and a plethora of research institutions, as well as pleasant residential zones. Not surprisingly, large swaths of nature are increasingly difficult to find and are accordingly cherished. Then there is southern Maryland and the Eastern Shore, both dominated by water. Mostly this means the Chesapeake Bay and its tributaries. But there's also the Atlantic Ocean, forming Maryland's eastern boundary.

Accordingly, I've separated the camping locations in this book by these distinct zones listed above. Virtually any Maryland resident can reach at least a few of the camping destinations in this book in a quick trip, certainly in less than an hour. Most of the state's population, like myself, is clustered in the central, urban zone. We can reach all of the book's destinations in less than four hours, and many, if not most, in less than three or even two.

In choosing which campgrounds to include, I tried very hard to keep in mind the "typical" camper, meaning in this case an amalgam of all the campers I met while doing research for this book. My personal preference is for out-of-the-way spots where you have to be fully self-sufficient, places where you can blissfully lose all the trappings of modernity for a few days. My bias for such places most probably comes through in my descriptions of the camping destinations such as the primitive sites in the state forests at Green Ridge, Potomac, and Garrett. However, I am aware that many more campers like easy access to facilities and don't want to travel too far or with too many jugs of potable water. Thus, I included many campgrounds that offer anything a camper could want. However,

I was careful to exclude campgrounds that were overrun with RVs and where finding silence and privacy were virtual impossibilities. Don't misunderstand, I've shared campground space with RVers and still enjoyed the experience immensely. Thus, a campground with a lot of RVs wasn't automatically excluded from this book. Besides, more and more campgrounds are geared toward catering to the RV set. But rest assured, you'll find many campgrounds in this book where RVs either aren't allowed or where their owners will find it impossible to reach.

THE OVERVIEW MAP AND OVERVIEW-MAP KEY

Use the overview map on the inside front cover to assess the exact location of each campground. The campground's number appears not only on the overview map but also on the map key facing the overview map, in the table of contents, and on the profile's first page.

The book is organized by region, as indicated in the table of contents. A map legend that details the symbols found on the campground layout maps appears on the inside back cover.

CAMPGROUND-LAYOUT MAPS

Each profile contains a detailed campground-layout map that provides an overhead look at campground sites, internal roads, facilities, and other key items. Each campground entrance's GPS coordinates are included with each profile.

GPS CAMPGROUND-ENTRANCE COORDINATES

Readers can easily access all campgrounds in this book by using the directions given and the overview map, which shows at least one major road leading into the area. But for those who enjoy using the latest GPS technology to navigate, the necessary data has been provided. This book includes the GPS coordinates for each campground. To collect accurate map data, each campground was recorded with a handheld GPS unit. Data collected was then downloaded and plotted onto a digital USGS topo map. More accurately known as UTM coordinates, the numbers index a specific point using a grid method. The survey datum used to arrive at the coordinates is NAD27. For readers who own a GPS unit, whether handheld or onboard a vehicle, the Universal Transverse Mercator (UTM) coordinates provided with each campground description may be entered into the GPS unit. Just make sure your GPS unit is set to navigate using the UTM system in conjunction with NAD27 datum.

One note about campground entries with multiple camping options, such as the C&O Canal sites and the South Mountain/Appalachian Trail sites: in these cases, I give the GPS data for the first camping site within that particular entry. For example, for the C&O Canal: Drive-in Sites, there are five campgrounds. I describe each in turn, moving in a northwesterly direction. Because Antietam Creek is the first described, the GPS information for the entire entry corresponds to the Antietam Creek site.

UTM COORDINATES: ZONE, EASTING, AND NORTHING

Within the UTM coordinates box in each campground description, there are three numbers labeled zone, easting, and northing. Here is an example from Fort Frederick State Park.

UTM Zone (NAD27) 17S
Easting 756861
Northing 4388136

The zone number (17) refers to one of the 60 longitudinal zones (vertical) of a map using the UTM projection. Each zone is 6° wide. The zone letter (S) refers to one of the 20 latitudinal zones (horizontal) that span from 80° South to 84° North.

The easting number (756861) references in meters how far east the point is from the zero value for eastings, which runs north-south through Greenwich, England. Increasing easting coordinates on a topo map or on your GPS screen indicate you are moving east; decreasing easting coordinates indicate you are moving west. Since lines of longitude converge at the poles, they are not parallel as lines of latitude are. This means that the distance between Full Easting Coordinates is 1,000 meters near the equator but becomes smaller as you travel farther north or south; the difference is small enough to be ignored, but only until you reach the polar regions.

In the Northern Hemisphere, the northing number (4388136) references in meters how far you are from the equator. Above the equator, northing coordinates increase by 1,000 meters between each parallel line of latitude (east-west lines). On a topo map or GPS receiver, increasing northing numbers indicate you are traveling north.

In the Southern Hemisphere, the northing number references how far you are from a latitude line that is 10 million meters south of the equator. Below the equator, northing coordinates decrease by 1,000 meters between each line of latitude. On a topo map, decreasing northing coordinates indicate you are traveling south.

THE RATING SYSTEM

This book rates each campground in six different categories, assigning from anywhere between one and five stars. There wasn't one campground that didn't have at least something special going for it. The real gems are the ones that have high rankings in five or all six categories. Of course, my rankings are subjective and largely dependent upon my specific experiences. However, I was careful to question other campers and especially rangers and employees to try and get a much fuller and objective view of each campground. Look at the rankings carefully, but don't exclude a campground solely upon a low ranking in one or more category. A campground with smallish campsites, for example, might very well lay in close proximity to an awe-inspiring view.

BEAUTY This category includes the area that extends beyond the campground itself. Easy access to thick forest, clear streams, or stupendous views gives a campground a high ranking, regardless of whether the specific sites themselves are apt to awe you.

PRIVACY This category refers to the ease with which campers in the next site can hear you and vice versa. Few campgrounds in this book don't offer at least a small green buffer between sites, but the ranking in this category will give you a good idea of how much.

SPACIOUSNESS Spaciousness refers to the physical dimensions of the campsites. If you are in a group, for example, this may be a top concern.

QUIET This is a difficult category to measure because different times of the year, times of the week, and luck of the neighborly draw will determine your experience. However, as indicated previously, I made every effort to talk with other campers and rangers/employees at each campground to try to get a fair sense of what one can expect any time of the year.

SECURITY DNR-run campgrounds are invariably very safe. Almost all have a camp host and easy access to ranger offices. Park police regularly patrol state campgrounds as well. I wouldn't predict much trouble at any of the campgrounds in this book. However, I gave some of the very remote campgrounds a lower rating for safety simply because there might well be no one around to deter crime. Thus, you will be more vulnerable. Of course, this isolation is what attracts me most about these places.

CLEANLINESS This is self-explanatory but refers to the amount of litter you might find at the campground. Overflowing trash cans, and restrooms that didn't look terribly well maintained were cause for knocking off a few stars in this category.

FIRST-AID KIT

A useful first-aid kit may contain more items than you might think necessary. These are just the basics. Prepackaged kits in waterproof bags (Atwater Carey and Adventure Medical make them) are available. As a preventive measure, take along sunscreen and insect repellent. Even though quite a few items are listed here, they pack down into a small space:

Ace bandages or Spenco joint wraps

Adhesive bandages, such as Band-Aids

Antibiotic ointment (Neosporin or the generic equivalent)

Antiseptic or disinfectant, such as Betadine or hydrogen peroxide

Aspirin or acetaminophen

Benadryl or the generic equivalent, diphenhydramine (in case of allergic reactions)

Butterfly-closure bandages

Epinephrine in a prefilled syringe (for people known to have severe allergic reactions to such things as bee stings)

Gauze (one roll)

Gauze compress pads (six 4- x 4-inch pads)

Matches or pocket lighter

Moleskin/Spenco "Second Skin"

Waterproof first-aid tape

Whistle (it's more effective in signaling rescuers than your voice)

ANIMAL AND PLANT HAZARDS

SNAKES Generally speaking, the prospect of being bitten by a snake should never deter a camper in Maryland. The state has only two native poisonous snakes: northern copperheads, which you may see in central, southern, and eastern Maryland, and timber rattlers, which live in the mountainous, western part of the state. Although the chances of being bitten by a snake are slim, take proper caution. For good information on snakes in Maryland, visit: **www.dnr.state.md.us/wildlife/vsnakes.asp.**

TICKS All outdoor recreationists in Maryland should be concerned about ticks. Your best protection is to be vigilant: Check yourself frequently and look hard. Often, the smaller the tick, the greater the chance for subsequent serious health problems. Tiny deer ticks (black-legged ticks), for example, carry Lyme disease; if you see a bull's-eye rash radiating from a tender red spot, see a doctor right away. If you experience flulike symptoms (intense malaise, fever, chills, and a headache) a day or two after camping, look very hard for the telltale bull's-eye rash and see a doctor to alleviate any concerns. If you find a tick attached to your skin, gently remove it with tweezers, taking care to pull it off gently so the mouthpart does not break off and remain attached. In general, ticks pose a major threat only during the warmest months of summer, but an unseasonably mild spring and/or warm autumn can mean a solid six or seven months of tick season. So take precautionary measures, but don't let it keep you inside your tent. *Note:* Lyme disease tends to be overdiagnosed and afflicts relatively few people.

POISON IVY The old maxim for poison ivy holds true: "Leaves of three, let it be." Poison sumac, however, can contain anywhere from 7 to 13 leaves. Since I am extremely allergic to poison ivy, I always take the following cautions: I do not scratch anything under any circumstances; if poison ivy is sitting on the skin, scratching and then touching skin anywhere else is the surest way of spreading it. I always carry alcohol-based moist towelettes, and at the end of the day, I rub my legs gently with the towelettes to stave off infection until I can get home and shower. (*Note:* It is very important that these moist towelettes contain alcohol. If they contain just soap, wiping with them will only move the poison ivy oil, urushiol, around, increasing the risk of infection.)

MOSQUITOES Many of the campgrounds in Southern Maryland and Eastern Shore are simply inundated with mosquitoes in the humid summer months. Protect yourself against mosquito bites by applying an effective repellent. Most people reach for repellents that contain DEET, which is fairly toxic stuff. I recently took Burt's Bees natural insect repellent with me on a trip into the Amazon jungle and found it very effective. Unlike DEET-based repellents, there is no maximum on the amount and frequency of use for Burt's.

The Asian Tiger mosquito, which spreads the West Nile virus, has been seen in Maryland, especially in places with lots of water. Even though West Nile has understandably grabbed headlines in recent years, your chances of contracting it are extraordinarily slim, and even if you do contract it, a reasonably healthy person who receives medical treatment will be able to stave off the disease's most-damaging effects.

RESOURCES

As you read this book, you'll see that the vast majority of the campgrounds are run by the Maryland Department of Natural Resources. I found time and time again that state-operated campgrounds were invariably clean, safe, and beautifully maintained. The Maryland DNR maintains an excellent Web site with links to all of the DNR-operated campgrounds featured in this book (33 of the 50). Visit **www.dnr.state.md.us/ outdoors/camping** for all the latest information and links. For information on private campgrounds in Maryland (including many not featured in this book), contact the Maryland Association of Campgrounds at (301) 271-7012, or visit **www.gocamping america.com/maryland.**

TIPS FOR A HAPPY CAMPING TRIP

There is nothing worse than a bad camping trip, especially because it is so easy to have a great time. To assist with making your outing a happy one, here are some pointers:

- **RESERVE YOUR SITE AHEAD OF TIME,** especially if it's a weekend or a holiday, or if the campground is wildly popular. Many prime campgrounds require at least a six-month lead time on reservations. Check before you go.

- **PICK YOUR CAMPING BUDDIES WISELY.** A family trip is pretty straightforward, but you may want to reconsider including grumpy Uncle Fred, who doesn't like bugs, sunshine, or marshmallows. After you know who's going, make sure that everyone is on the same page regarding expectations of difficulty (amenities or the lack thereof, physical exertion, and so on), sleeping arrangements, and food requirements.

- **DON'T DUPLICATE EQUIPMENT SUCH AS COOKING POTS** and lanterns among campers in your party. Carry what you need to have a good time, but don't turn the trip into a major moving experience.

- **DRESS FOR THE SEASON.** Educate yourself on the temperature highs and lows of the specific area you plan to visit. It may be warm at night in the summer in your backyard, but up in the mountains it will be quite chilly.

- **PITCH YOUR TENT ON A LEVEL SURFACE,** preferably one covered with leaves, pine straw, or grass. Use a tarp or specially designed footprint to thwart ground moisture and to protect the tent floor. Do a little site maintenance, such as picking up the small rocks and sticks that can damage your tent floor and make sleep uncomfortable. If you have a separate tent rain fly but don't think you'll need it, keep it rolled up at the base of the tent in case it starts raining at midnight.

- **IF YOU ARE NOT COMFORTABLE SLEEPING ON THE GROUND,** take a sleeping pad with you that is full-length and thicker than you think you might need. This will not only keep your hips from aching on hard ground, but will also help keep you warm. A wide range of thin, light, inflatable pads is available at camping stores today, and these are a much better choice than home air mattresses, which conduct heat away from the body and tend to deflate during the night.

- **IF YOU'RE NOT HIKING INTO A PRIMITIVE CAMPSITE,** there is no real need to skimp on food due to weight. Plan tasty meals and bring everything you will need to prepare, cook, eat, and clean up.

- **IF YOU TEND TO USE THE BATHROOM MULTIPLE TIMES AT NIGHT,** you should plan ahead. Leaving a warm sleeping bag and stumbling around in the dark to find the restroom, whether it be a pit toilet, a fully plumbed comfort station, or just the woods, is not fun. Keep a flashlight and any other accoutrements you may need by the tent door and know exactly where to head in the dark.

- **STANDING DEAD TREES AND STORMDAMAGED LIVING TREES** can pose a real hazard to tent campers. These trees may have loose or broken limbs that could fall at any time. When choosing a campsite or even just a spot to rest during a hike, look up.

CAMPING ETIQUETTE

Camping experiences can vary wildly depending on a variety of factors, such as weather, preparedness, fellow campers, and time of year. Here are a few tips on how to create good vibes with fellow campers and wildlife you encounter.

- **OBTAIN ALL PERMITS AND AUTHORIZATION AS REQUIRED.** Make sure you check in, pay your fee, and mark your site as directed. Don't make the mistake of grabbing a seemingly empty site that looks more appealing than your site. It could be reserved. If you're unhappy with the site you've selected, check with the campground host for other options.

- **LEAVE ONLY FOOTPRINTS.** Be sensitive to the ground beneath you. Be sure to place all garbage in designated receptacles or pack it out if none is available. No one likes to see the trash someone else has left behind.

- **NEVER SPOOK ANIMALS.** It's common for animals to wander through campsites, where they may be accustomed to the presence of humans (and our food). An unannounced approach, a sudden movement, or a loud noise startles most animals. A surprised animal can be dangerous to you, to others, and to themselves. Give them plenty of space.

- **PLAN AHEAD.** Know your equipment, your ability, and the area where you are camping—and prepare accordingly. Be self-sufficient at all times; carry necessary supplies for changes in weather or other conditions. A well-executed trip is a satisfaction to you and to others.

- **BE COURTEOUS TO OTHER CAMPERS,** hikers, bikers, and others you encounter. If you run into the owner of a large RV, don't panic. Just wave, feign eye contact, and then walk slowly away.

- **STRICTLY FOLLOW THE CAMPGROUND'S RULES** regarding the building of fires. Never burn trash. Trash smoke smells horrible, and trash debris in a fire pit or grill is unsightly.

VENTURING AWAY FROM THE CAMPGROUND

If you go for a hike, bike, or other excursion into the wilderness, here are some tips:

- **ALWAYS CARRY FOOD AND WATER,** whether you are planning to go overnight or not. Food will give you energy, help keep you warm, and sustain you in an emergency until help arrives. Bring potable water or treat water by boiling or filtering before drinking from a lake or stream.

- **STAY ON DESIGNATED TRAILS.** Most hikers get lost when they leave the trail. Even on the most clearly marked trails, there is usually a point where you have to stop and consider which direction to head. If you become disoriented, don't panic. As soon as you think you may be off-track, stop, assess your current direction, and then retrace your steps back to the point where you went awry. If you have absolutely no idea how to continue, return to the trailhead the way you came in. Should you become completely lost and have no idea of how to return to the trailhead, remaining in place along the trail and waiting for help is most often the best option for adults and always the best option for children.

- **BE ESPECIALLY CAREFUL WHEN CROSSING STREAMS.** Whether you are fording the stream or crossing on a log, make every step count. If you have any doubt about maintaining your balance on a log, go ahead and ford the stream instead. When fording a stream, use a trekking pole or stout stick for balance and face upstream as you cross. If a stream seems too deep to ford, turn back. Whatever is on the other side is not worth risking your life.

- **BE CAREFUL AT OVERLOOKS.** Although these areas may provide spectacular views, they are potentially hazardous. Stay back from the edge of outcrops and be absolutely sure of your footing: a misstep can mean a nasty and possibly fatal fall.

- **KNOW THE SYMPTOMS OF HYPOTHERMIA.** Shivering and forgetfulness are the two most common indicators of this insidious killer. Hypothermia can occur at any elevation, even in the summer. Wearing cotton clothing puts you especially at risk, because cotton, when wet, wicks heat away from the body. To prevent hypothermia, dress in layers using synthetic clothing for insulation, use a cap and gloves to reduce heat loss, and protect yourself with waterproof, breathable outerwear. If symptoms arise, get the victim to shelter, a fire, hot liquids, and dry clothes or a dry sleeping bag.

- **TAKE ALONG YOUR BRAIN.** A cool, calculating mind is the single most important piece of equipment you'll ever need on the trail. Think before you act. Watch your step. Plan ahead. Avoiding accidents before they happen is the best recipe for a rewarding and relaxing hike.

WESTERN MARYLAND

01
BIG RUN
STATE PARK

AT 300 ACRES, BIG RUN STATE PARK is relatively modest in size, but it sits within the Savage River State Forest, which, at 53,000 acres, is the largest of Maryland's state forests and parks. Big Run is just one of the many state parks and forests in Garrett County; what sets it apart from its neighbors is its proximity to the unspoiled Savage River Reservoir, where anglers can fish for a seemingly endless supply of bass, catfish, crappie, perch, trout, and walleye. Canoe rentals are offered at BJ's store just north of the state park, on Big Run Road.

Another feature that distinguishes Big Run from its larger park neighbor, New Germany, is that camping here is year-round. Because of the cold and the threat of heavy snow, winter camping is largely a private experience. The numerous hiking trails in the state forest provide for some great cross-country skiing.

If you've brought a boat, you'll want to snag one of the sites in the 80s or sites 78, 79, or 90, which are closest to the boat launch for the reservoir. These are fairly big sites, but they sit more or less in the open, away from forest canopy.

If you are more interested in the surrounding forest and its hiking trails, go for the sites north of the boat launch, off Big Run Road (sites 60 through 77). One word of warning: Sites 76 and 77 are very close to one another; they even seem to share space. If you're a small group that exceeds the limit for one site, 76 and 77 might actually be good to grab for their proximity to one another.

> *Big Run is just one of the many state parks and forests in Garrett County; what sets it apart from its neighbors is its proximity to the unspoiled Savage River Reservoir.*

RATINGS

Beauty: ✿ ✿ ✿ ✿
Privacy: ✿ ✿ ✿
Quiet: ✿ ✿ ✿
Spaciousness: ✿ ✿ ✿ ✿
Security: ✿ ✿ ✿ ✿ ✿
Cleanliness: ✿ ✿ ✿ ✿ ✿

ADDRESS:	**Big Run State Park c/o New Germany State Park 349 Headquarters Lane Grantsville, MD 21536 (301) 895-5453**
OPERATED BY:	**Maryland Department of Natural Resources**
OPEN:	**All year**
SITES:	**30**
EACH SITE HAS:	**Picnic table, fire grill, lantern post**
ASSIGNMENT:	**First come, first served**
REGISTRATION:	**Through New Germany State Park, (301) 895-5453, or self-register at information desk in Big Run State Park**
FACILITIES:	**Picnic pavilion, restroom, water**
PARKING:	**2 vehicles max. per site**
FEE:	**$15/night; group site (25 people max.), $60/night**
RESTRICTIONS:	*Pets:* **Allowed on a leash** *Quiet Hours:* **11 p.m.– 7 a.m.** *Visitors:* **Max. 6 people per site** *Fires:* **In fire rings** *Alcohol:* **At site only** *Stay Limit:* **2 weeks** *Other:* **Check-out is 3 p.m.**

The 6-mile Monroe Run Trail commences from between sites 62 and 64, and these sites, along with 65 and 67, could very well be the most pleasurable spots to have. They sit in the forested sections of the park, away from the main camp roads. The trail follows the Monroe Run into nearby New Germany State Park (see page 69). The trail shouldn't be missed; it's a modest 6 miles, but it winds through pristine forests and over innumerable streams. It guarantees a workout, but it's very lovely.

In all, you really can't go wrong in Big Run; it's fairly small, so there's really not a whole lot of action, company, or noise. And if you want an even more rustic camping experience, you can head straight north on Big Run Road or east on Savage River Road for loads of camping opportunities in the Savage River State Forest (see page 81).

MAP

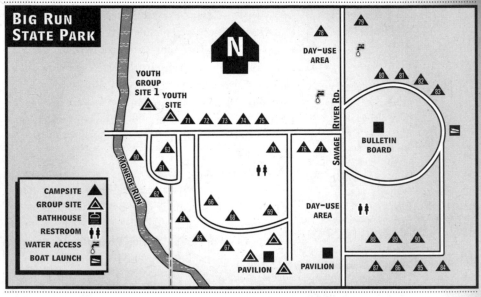

GETTING THERE

Take Exit 22 off I-68 and
follow Chestnut Ridge Road
south to New Germany
Road. Pass New Germany
State Park headquarters
and take a left onto
Big Run Road.

GPS COORDINATES

UTM Zone (NAD27) 17S
Easting 659964
Northing 4378813

> *Brunswick Family Campground possesses some prime real estate, astride a particularly beautiful stretch of the Potomac River.*

BRUNSWICK IS A SMALL CITY (population 5,000) in southwestern Frederick County, near the Washington County border. It's on the National Register of Historic Places because of its importance in the early-to-mid-1900s as a railroading town. The city also bumps up against the C&O Canal and the Potomac River. This wonderful location is what makes Brunswick Family Campground worth a visit. The campground itself used to be an airfield, so there's lots of space.

I must acknowledge, however, that I really debated whether or not I should include Brunswick Family Campground in this book. Of the 50 campgrounds I've described here, I might very well rank it last. First, it's primarily an RV campground. Second, while the grounds are well maintained, the basketball court and, more importantly, the bathhouse (only one on site), are not. So why did I decide ultimately to include it? Location, location, location.

Brunswick Family Campground possesses some prime real estate, astride a particularly beautiful stretch of the Potomac River. The same can be said of several other campsites in this book, most notably the C&O Canal drive-in and hiker/biker sites. However, the advantage that Brunswick Family Campground has over those is that you won't have to haul your gear to get there, and you're always assured of getting a spot (campground literature claims that there are 300 tent sites, which means they really pack them in). Plus, the campground is less than a mile down a dirt road from the center of town and its most notable attraction, the Brunswick Railroad Museum, which also houses the C&O Canal National Historic Park Visitor Center for nearby Canal Lock 30. Plus, the campground enjoys proximity to state parks; Civil War battlefields; and Harpers Ferry, West Virginia. As a result, it could

RATINGS

Beauty: ☆ ☆
Privacy: ☆
Spaciousness: ☆ ☆
Quiet: ☆ ☆ ☆
Security: ☆ ☆ ☆ ☆ ☆
Cleanliness: ☆ ☆ ☆

provide for a nice family outing. There is often musical entertainment on weekends, when the campground is full. Most of the campers are locals, and Brunswick enjoys a reputation for friendliness.

My recommendation is to use the campground as a midweek destination for boating or fishing. (I visited on a gorgeous Tuesday in June, and the place was virtually empty.) There's a convenient boat ramp just beyond the entrance road.

The tent-only sites sit to the right of the entrance on Airport Drive, just beyond RV Section C. The farther you head to the right, the farther you get from the RVs. However, moving farther to the right also brings you closer to the waste-treatment plant that looms just over the campground boundary. If you get too close, you will most probably smell it. Thus, try to get a site closer to Section C so you won't see or smell the plant. Plus, this area is actually pretty nice; it's thickly wooded (though not very private).

There is one tent site that is absolutely fantastic, and if you can get it, your experience should be quite special. All the way to the left when you enter, beyond sites 1 through 20 in RV Section A, sits one tent site by itself in a little copse right in front of the river, with a small path heading off to the woods on the left. It's very private and very spacious. It's one of the nicest spots you'll get anywhere, not just in this campground. There are other tent sites that aren't bad, either, though across the campground from the river. They are just to the left of the basketball court when you enter, toward the tree line.

KEY INFORMATION

ADDRESS:	Brunswick Family Campground Maple Avenue Brunswick, MD 21716 (301) 834-8050
OPERATED BY:	City of Brunswick, MD
OPEN:	First weekend in April–last weekend in November
SITES:	365 (300 tent, 65 RV)
EACH SITE HAS:	Fire ring, picnic table
ASSIGNMENT:	Reservations recommended, accepted after January 1 for that calendar year
REGISTRATION:	(301) 834-8050
FACILITIES:	Ball fields, bathhouse, boat ramp, dumping station, playground, vending
PARKING:	In designated areas
FEE:	Friday and Saturday, $25/night ($31/night electric); Sunday–Thursday, $20/night ($25 electric); 15% discount for disabled, over 60, and military persons
RESTRICTIONS:	*Pets:* On a leash *Quiet Hours:* 10 p.m.–8 a.m. *Visitors:* Requested to stop by office and sign in *Fires:* In fire pits *Alcohol:* Not permitted *Stay Limit:* 2 weeks; campers can come back after 7 days *Other:* Check-out is 2 p.m.

MAP

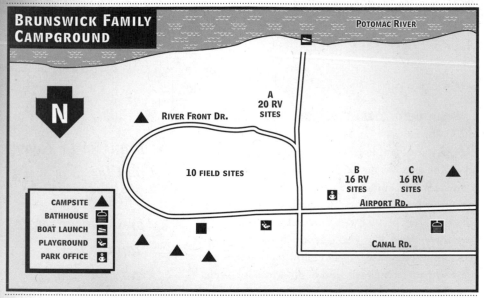

BRUNSWICK FAMILY CAMPGROUND

POTOMAC RIVER

N

RIVER FRONT DR.

A
20 RV SITES

10 FIELD SITES

B
16 RV SITES

C
16 RV SITES

AIRPORT RD.

CANAL RD.

CAMPSITE
BATHHOUSE
BOAT LAUNCH
PLAYGROUND
PARK OFFICE

GETTING THERE

From Frederick, take I-70 to US Route 340 West to Exit 2, MD 17 South. Take A Street over the railroad tracks and then head left on the dirt road.

GPS COORDINATES

UTM Zone (NAD27) 18S
Easting 274562
Northing 4354126

03 CATOCTIN MOUNTAIN PARK

CATOCTIN MOUNTAIN PARK has a pedigreed history as a getaway spot—the presidential retreat at Camp David lies on the same property. The area was developed in the 1930s partly as a retreat for the families of federal employees. Although people are still fond of saying that D.C.'s population changes every election year and that no one actually *lives* there, those of us who grew up in and around D.C. know otherwise. We also know that summer—a time when it feels like the rest of the world is coming into the city—can be brutally hot and humid. After all, the city was built on a swamp. Thus, a place like Catoctin, not too far away even in those days before mass transport and reliable, paved roads, is truly a wonderful retreat.

Franklin D. Roosevelt was the first to use Catoctin as a presidential getaway, in 1942. He named it "Shangri-La." When Roosevelt died, there was some controversy over whether the land would remain in federal hands or revert to Maryland state parkland. A compromise was reached whereby the land north of Route 77 would remain under federal control, while that south would go back to Maryland. (This southern area is now Cunningham Falls State Park; see profile on page 33.) The deal became official in 1954, and then president Eisenhower renamed the retreat after his grandson.

Obviously, a visitor to Catoctin Park shouldn't expect to be able to do any snooping around Camp David. In fact, chances are, you won't even know where it is in relation to where you're hiking or camping. (That said, I've been camping here when helicopters busily ferried dignitaries to and from the retreat). The sections of the park that aren't off-limits contain more than 5,800 acres and more than 25 miles of hiking trails. Adding adjacent Cunningham

> *Franklin D. Roosevelt was the first to use Catoctin as a presidential getaway, naming it 'Shangri-La.'*

RATINGS

Beauty: ✿ ✿ ✿ ✿ ✿
Privacy: ✿ ✿ ✿ ✿
Spaciousness: ✿ ✿ ✿
Quiet: ✿ ✿ ✿ ✿
Security: ✿ ✿ ✿ ✿ ✿
Cleanliness: ✿ ✿ ✿ ✿ ✿

ADDRESS: Catoctin Mountain
Park
6602 Foxville Road
Thurmont, MD
21788-1598
(301) 663-9388
or: National Park
Service, c/o Harpers
Ferry Center
P.O. Box 50
Harpers Ferry, WV
25425

OPERATED BY: National Park
Service

OPEN: April 15–third Sun-
day in November

SITES: 51

EACH SITE HAS: Picnic table, grill,
lantern post, tent
pad

ASSIGNMENT: First come, first
served

REGISTRATION: Self-register at
headquarters near
entrance

FACILITIES: Bathhouses

PARKING: Only 1 vehicle at
individual site,
very limited
overflow parking

FEE: $20/night

RESTRICTIONS: *Pets:* On a leash
Quiet Hours: 10 p.m.–
6 a.m.
Visitors: Max. 5
people or the
immediate house-
hold per site
Fires: In fire rings
Alcohol: Not allowed
Stay Limit: No more
than 7 consecutive
days, or 14 days in
a year
Other: Max. tent size
9 by 12 feet

Falls State Park, there's no shortage of recreational opportunities.

Catoctin's Owens Creek Campground sits near its namesake, the clean and clear Owens Creek. Several hiking trails also come quite close, including the Catoctin Trail, which runs all the way through the park, into Cunningham Falls State Park, and farther south through the Frederick Municipal Forest. Nearer the park headquarters, it's easy to access trails that take in Chimney Rock, Wolf Rock, Thurmont Vista, and the Blue Ridge Summit Overlook, a fantastic loop through hardwood forests with grand, sweeping views.

I tend to have a bias toward the last site on any loop because of its minimal through traffic. For Catoctin, this means Site 30, which sits virtually by itself at the very end of the loop. If access to the bathhouse and water is most important, try to snag Site 10 or 20. But the sites nearest Owens Creek are the most popular, and justly so—it's a lovely little tributary, and the sites are very close to the creek. Essentially, the sites to the left of the entrance area—sites 1, 2, 4, 7, 14 to 16, 18, and 28 to 30—head toward the creek. Of these, sites 18, 28, and 29 are the best, with 30 a good bet as well because of its additional proximity to hiking trails.

Outside of the main campground loop, there are also two Adirondack shelters where you can camp. These shelters are free, but permits are required (obtainable at the visitor center, not reservable in advance). Tents must be set up inside the shelters. The shelters can accommodate five people and provide access to a pit toilet. They both sit within 3 miles of parking areas.

MAP

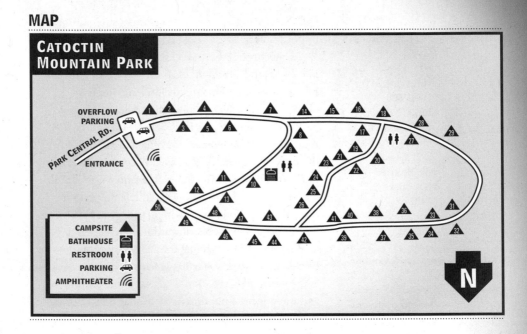

CATOCTIN MOUNTAIN PARK

OVERFLOW PARKING

Park Central Rd.

ENTRANCE

CAMPSITE
BATHHOUSE
RESTROOM
PARKING
AMPHITHEATER

N

From Frederick, take US Route 15 17 miles north to Thurmont. Take MD Route 77 West. Go 3 miles and turn right onto Park Central Road.

GPS COORDINATES

UTM Zone (NAD27) 18S
Easting 286203
Northing 4392118

> *All campsites along the canal have two things in common: the Potomac in front and the towpath behind.*

THE **C&O CANAL FOLLOWS** the Potomac River for 185 miles from Washington, D.C., to Cumberland, Maryland. It served for almost 100 years beginning in 1828, and a multitude of original structures still stand, attesting to its durability and workmanship. It came close to becoming a highway, but through the tireless efforts in the mid-1950s of Supreme Court Justice William O. Douglas, it was turned instead into a linear park in 1971. Today, we are the beneficiaries.

The C&O Canal enjoys a reputation as the best-preserved 19th-century canal in America, and restoration projects continue to this day. Potomac floods have the effect of washing away major portions of the canal, so restoration will probably go on perpetually. Like the monuments and museums in D.C., the canal's mission is a very public one. To that end, a whole series of hiker/biker campsites are set up and maintained and are free of charge (see the next three profiles in this book).

There are also five drive-in campsites along the C&O Canal, none of which have electric hookups. In choosing where to go and what to see along the canal, you have to familiarize yourself with the numbering system. Everything along the canal is assigned a number according to its distance from Mile 0, at the canal's starting point at the Georgetown Visitor's Center in Washington, D.C.

The five drive-in sites are spread along the canal but are more along the northwestern sections toward Cumberland (as opposed to southeast toward Washington). They are Antietam Creek (Mile 70), McCoys Ferry (Mile 110), Fifteen Mile Creek (Mile 141), Paw Paw (Mile 156), and Spring Gap (Mile 173).

All campsites along the canal have two things in common: the Potomac in front and the towpath behind. This means an endless supply of boating, fishing,

RATINGS

Beauty: ✫ ✫ ✫ ✫
Privacy: ✫ ✫
Quiet: ✫ ✫ ✫ ✫
Spaciousness: ✫ ✫ ✫ ✫
Security: ✫ ✫ ✫ ✫
Cleanliness: ✫ ✫ ✫ ✫

swimming, and hiking opportunities. Every site is somewhat different in character, however, in that the surrounding topography changes and nearby historical sites and towns (or lack thereof) change the experience of camping in each site. As a general rule, expect a large, cleared area with individual campsites scattered around the available space. While the sites are usually big, they're never terribly far from one another. Antietam Creek has as its main draw point its proximity to Antietam National Battlefield, which is a short drive (or canoe ride) away. Antietam is hallowed ground, site of the bloodiest battle in the Civil War. Excellent maintenance and educational opportunities distinguish the park. But it's also an exceedingly beautiful place, and a canoe or kayak trip upstream through the battlefield site is a special experience. From MD Route 40 in Boonsboro, take Route 34 West to Route 665 West (Harpers Ferry Road). There are 20 campsites at Antietam Creek, and water is available between mid-April and mid-November.

McCoys Ferry tends to be more popular, as it has RV parking. As mentioned previously, there are no electric sites at any of the C&O Canal campgrounds, but RVs in the area can use this parking lot. McCoys Ferry is also popular because it has a boat ramp for quick launch into the Potomac. The launch parking lot is where you have to leave your car. Be aware that there is no potable water at this site. McCoys Ferry has 14 sites and is nicely situated just south of Fort Frederick State Park (see page 42) and Big Pool. To reach McCoys Ferry, take I-70 to Exit 12 and follow MD Route 56 past Big Pool and Fort Frederick. Take a right onto McCoys Ferry Rd.

Fifteen Mile Creek, with ten sites, also has parking and a boat launch. There is water available between mid-April and mid-November. If you need other supplies, the town of Little Orleans is nearby. The campsite sits on the southern edge of Green Ridge State Forest (see page 54), so if the level terrain of the canal gets tiresome, you can head for the forested hills. A bit farther out, back on I-68, is the Sideling Hill Visitor Center. The four-story center sits perched atop one of the most dramatic rock exposures in the eastern U.S.

ADDRESS:	C&O Canal NHP Headquarters 1850 Dual Highway, Suite 100 Hagerstown, MD 21740-6620 (301) 739-4200
OPERATED BY:	National Park Service
OPEN:	All year
SITES:	5 locations, 71 sites total
EACH SITE HAS:	Picnic table, fire pit
ASSIGNMENT:	First come, first served
REGISTRATION:	Self-registration at each site, pay before occupying site
FACILITIES:	Chemical toilets, grills, water (except McCoys Ferry)
PARKING:	Max. 2 vehicles per site; park only at designated sites, never on grass
FEE:	$10/night
RESTRICTIONS:	*Pets:* On a leash or under control *Quiet Hours:* 10 p.m.– 6 a.m. *Visitors:* Max. 8 people or 2 tents per site *Fires:* In grills or fire rings only *Stay Limit:* Total of 30 days for the calendar year, only 14 of which can be consecutive or between May 1 and October 1

MAP

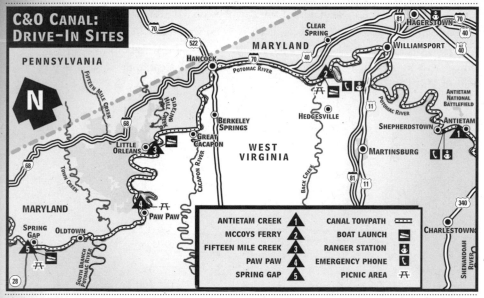

C&O CANAL: DRIVE-IN SITES

ANTIETAM CREEK	▲1	CANAL TOWPATH
MCCOYS FERRY	▲2	BOAT LAUNCH
FIFTEEN MILE CREEK	▲3	RANGER STATION
PAW PAW	▲4	EMERGENCY PHONE
SPRING GAP	▲5	PICNIC AREA

GETTING THERE

Varies; see text.

GPS COORDINATES

UTM Zone (NAD27) 18S
Easting 263635
Northing 4366789

The highway blasted through the mountain exposed almost 850 feet of vertical rock layers formed some 350 million years ago. To reach Fifteen Mile Creek, take I-68 to MD Route 68 (Orleans Road) to the town of Little Orleans.

Paw Paw may very well be the canal's most popular site. The chief attraction here is the Paw Paw Tunnel, a 3,100-foot-long tunnel constructed between 1836 and 1850. Paw Paw allows easy access to Green Ridge State Forest, entering from the west side. Paw Paw campground, with eight sites, is loaded with amenities. Aside from parking and a boat launch, there are picnic areas, phones, and a camp store and restaurants nearby, just across the bridge in the town of Paw Paw, West Virginia. To reach the Paw Paw camping area, head north from Little Orleans on Orleans Road (see directions to Fifteen Mile Creek above), pick up Old-town Road in the Green Ridge State Forest to MD Route 51, and head south.

The amenities listed for Paw Paw are also found at Spring Gap (sans the restaurants), the westernmost drive-in campground, with 19 sites. This is a more remote section of the canal, sitting in the shadow of

Warrior Mountain (what a great name!) and within 10 miles of the canal's terminus at Cumberland. To reach it, head north from Paw Paw on MD Route 51 to the town of Spring Gap; the campsite is just beyond. There is no water here.

Note: Group sites can hold up to 35, require advanced reservations (call the park office), and are located at Marsden Tract (Mile 11) and adjacent to the drive-in site at Fifteen Mile Creek (Mile 141).

05
C&O CANAL:
HIKER/BIKER CAMPSITES FROM SWAIN'S LOCK (MILE 16.6) TO KILLIANSBURG CAVE (MILE 75.2)

> *In virtually every case, the campsites sit along the Potomac and the C&O in wooded copses.*

THERE ARE 32 TENT-ONLY HIKER-BIKER campsites along the canal, located roughly every 5 miles. The H/B sites are limited to one night per site. This can be an annoyance for a lot of people, as it requires breaking down and cleaning up daily. However, it creates a great situation for people who want to hike, bike, or boat their way along a segment of the river and canal. My buddy Jack and I kayaked from Paw Paw, West Virginia, down to Hancock, Maryland, and the campsites along the way were perfectly suited for our needs.

While the H/B sites are often physically indistinguishable from one another, what should determine which you want comes down to location: in virtually every case, they sit along the Potomac and the C&O in wooded copses. What I mean here about location is distance from wherever you're traveling and distance from where you'll have to leave your car. In some cases, there's a hike required to get to the site from the parking area. This has an advantage in that the farther you go, the greater the chances of solitude. Of course, if you're hauling a lot of gear, it might be nice to have a quick walk from the car to the site.

Be aware that the C&O Canal is popular in many places; you should expect hikers and bikers passing by your site at all hours of the day. This leaves some people a bit skittish in that their belongings are easily accessed by others walking by while the camper is, say, out on the river. This is a legitimate concern. However, I've never spoken to one camper who has had an experience of thievery while camping along the C&O Canal (and this includes myself).

Officially, swimming is prohibited in the canal, as well as in the Potomac where it borders D.C. and Montgomery County. (This means everything south of Indian Flats H/B site—as for this entry, it covers Swains Lock,

RATINGS

Beauty: ✿ ✿ ✿ ✿
Privacy: ✿ ✿ ✿ ✿
Quiet: ✿ ✿ ✿ ✿
Spaciousness: ✿ ✿ ✿ ✿ ✿
Security: ✿ ✿ ✿ ✿
Cleanliness: ✿ ✿ ✿ ✿

Horsepen Branch, Chisel Branch, Turtle Run, and Marble Quarry—so if swimming in the river is your primary goal in camping along the canal, head farther north. That includes Indian Flats, Calico Rocks, Bald Eagle Island, Huckleberry Hill, and Killiansburg Cave in this entry and all the other sites in the following two entries in this book). The Park Service doesn't recommend swimming anywhere in the river, as the currents can be deceptively strong. However, swimming near the shore and taking due caution is generally safe.

One last word about the H/B sites; generally speaking, each site is just one cleared area where folks can pitch a tent. The amount of cleared space corresponds to the popularity of the area. The first H/B site is at Mile 16.6, at Swains Lock. This is a very popular area, with phones, food, and bike and boat rentals nearby. There's a lot of camping space here, as this could be the most heavily trafficked area on the entire canal. A major reason for that is Great Falls, 2.5 miles downstream. Great Falls is a beautiful place and the best place to see the Potomac at its most awesome as it roils through serrated rocks. It's also popular with hikers taking on the Billy Goat Trail and exploring Mather Gorge. To get to Swains Lock, take I-495 to River Road West (Exit 39) and then turn left about a quarter mile past Piney Meetinghouse Road.

Horsepen Branch H/B (Mile 26.1) sits right on the edge of the McKee-Beshers Wildlife Management Area (2,000 acres) and is just north of Seneca Creek State Park (6,300 acres). Between the two of them, hikers have it good. From I-270, use MD 109 south, and take West Willard Road until it ends at Sycamore Landing. You can park at the boat launch there and then walk south (downstream) for 1 mile.

Chisel Branch (Mile 30.5) is where things begin to feel a bit more remote; the day crowds dry up and there's a better sense of wildness. Follow the directions above to Horsepen Branch, but on West Willard Road, take a right toward Edwards Ferry and park there. The H/B campsite is 0.3 miles upstream. The lockhouse just upstream at Edwards Ferry (1791 to 1836) is still in great condition.

KEY INFORMATION

ADDRESS: C&O Canal NHP Headquarters 1850 Dual Highway, Suite 100 Hagerstown, MD 21740-6620 (301) 739-4200

OPERATED BY: National Park Service

OPEN: All H/B sites open year-round

SITES: 10

EACH SITE HAS: Grill, chemical toilet, picnic table, and pump well water. (I did once have occasion when the pump didn't work, so it's not a bad idea to plan for that possibility.)

ASSIGNMENT: First come, first served

REGISTRATION: None

FACILITIES: Varies by site; see text

PARKING: Vehicles must be left at the nearest parking area; see text for individual sites

FEE: Free

RESTRICTIONS: *Pets:* None
Quiet Hours: None
Visitors: Max. 8 people per site
Fires: In fire rings or portable grills only
Alcohol: Not allowed
Stay Limit: 1 night per site, per trip
Other: Only dead wood only can be collected for fires

MAP

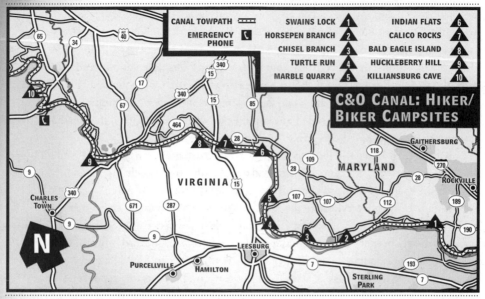

CANAL TOWPATH	▦	SWAINS LOCK	1	INDIAN FLATS	6
EMERGENCY PHONE	☎	HORSEPEN BRANCH	2	CALICO ROCKS	7
		CHISEL BRANCH	3	BALD EAGLE ISLAND	8
		TURTLE RUN	4	HUCKLEBERRY HILL	9
		MARBLE QUARRY	5	KILLIANSBURG CAVE	10

C&O CANAL: HIKER/ BIKER CAMPSITES

GETTING THERE

Varies; see text.

GPS COORDINATES

UTM Zone (NAD27) 18S
Easting 292752
Northing 4327160

Turtle Run (Mile 34.4): this area is studded with culverts (no less than seven of them within a 2-mile span). Things go, temporarily, back to feeling a bit like they did closer to D.C. Because White's Ferry is still operating, this area attracts a lot of visitors. Take MD 109 to a right onto MD 107 North. Turtle Run is 1 mile south of MD 107.

MD 107 leads to a toll ferry across the river to Leesburg, VA. You can park at the ferry and then walk downstream 1.1 miles to Turtle Run. Marble Quarry (Mile 38.2) is similar to Turtle Run, only upstream instead of down. To get there, park at White's Ferry.

Indian Flats H/B (Mile 42.5) is the first campsite where you are legally allowed to swim in the Potomac. Indian Flats sits roughly equidistant from two boat launches at Monocacy downstream and Nolands Ferry upstream. Use MD 109 south to MD 28 west toward Monocacy and head to the parking at the Monocacy Aqueduct. Indian Flats is 0.3 miles upstream. The Monocacy Aqueduct is something to see in and of itself. Described by the NPS as "An Icon of American Civil Engineering," it is the largest of the canal's aqueducts and is considered an engineering marvel.

Calico Rocks H/B (Mile 47.6) is next. A word of warning about this site: an operable railroad is very close by, and it can get noisy, even during the night. From Frederick, take Rt. 340 to Rt. 15 to Point of Rocks. The Calico Rocks H/B is 0.5 miles downstream. The same issue with rail noise plagues the next H/B site: Bald Eagle Island (Mile 50.3). Follow the same directions for Calico Rocks, but take MD 464 west to a left on Lander Road and park there. Bald Eagle Island H/B is 0.6 miles downstream. One potentially positive thing that both Calico Rocks and Bald Eagle Island share is their close proximity to both Frederick and Brunswick; if you needed any supplies or wanted to eat (or if the weather is atrocious), it's a quick and easy trip to civilization.

Between Bald Eagle Island and the next H/B site, there's a big gap; this is filled by the city of Brunswick, the Appalachian Trail as it heads down South Mountain (in fact, the AT and the canal towpath are one and the same between Lock 31 and 32), and the river crossing for Harpers Ferry, where the Potomac and the Shenandoah rivers meet. Mile 62.9 is where you'll find Huckleberry Hill H/B. This, like Seneca to the south, is a popular spot, mostly because of its proximity to Harpers Ferry. One word of warning here: if you've come for boating, the waters just downstream, between Locks 32 and 34, are considered very hazardous. Take MD 34 from Boonsboro to a left on Harpers Ferry Road, crossing through Antietam, and follow the river south to Dargan. Park at Dargan Bend and then walk 2 miles downstream.

Last is Killiansburg Cave (Mile 75.2), so called because of the small caves in the rock where locals sought shelter during the battle of Antietam. (In between is the Antietam Creek Drive-in Campsite, see page 20). Proximity to Antietam National Battlefield and a Ranger Station just downstream make Killiansburg a nice camping spot. Take MD 34 from Boonsboro, cross Rt. 65 at Sharpsburg, and take the first right toward the boat launch at Snyders Landing. Killiansburg Cave is approximately 1 mile downstream.

Cacapon Junction is the area where the Cacapon River, a favorite Potomac tributary, meets the Potomac on the West Virginia side.

FOR GENERAL INFORMATION on hiker/biker sites, read the introductory material in the previous profile. What follows is a continuation of those sites, moving northwesterly along the C&O Canal toward Cumberland.

After Antietam and Killiansburg Cave comes Horseshoe Bend hiker/biker site (Mile 79.2). From Hagerstown, Take MD 65 South to a right at Taylors Landing boat launch. Horseshoe Bend is 1.7 miles downstream. This area is closest to the city of Hagerstown, where you can get whatever supplies you need.

Big Woods (Mile 82.7) has parking 1.6 miles downstream at Taylors Landing ramp. From either Hagerstown or Sharpsburg, take MD 65 to Taylors Landing. Also, the canal's midpoint is here, just before the next hiker/biker site, Opequon Junction and Lock 43. Big Woods hiker/biker campsite enjoys a reputation for privacy, as it sits down a little trail from the canal towpath, while most others sit just off the towpath. Between Big Woods and the next upstream launch at Big Slackwater, at roughly Mile 87, major erosion and damage from flooding have rendered portions of the towpath impassable. There are detour instructions, and work is ongoing to repair the trail, but be aware.

Opequon Junction (Mile 90.9) has parking 2 miles downstream at McMahons Mill. To get there from I-70, take Exit 28 on MD 632 West. For the next hiker/biker site, Cumberland Valley (Mile 95.2), park 4.1 miles downstream at Williamsport, which has a visitor center, boat and bike rental, phone, picnic area, food, and a boat launch. Williamsport itself is worth a look around. Most Marylanders like to boast that Annapolis was once the national capital and is still America's oldest continuous state capital. But few Marylanders are aware that tiny Williamsport was once considered for the national capital by none other than George Washington

RATINGS

Beauty: ✿ ✿ ✿ ✿
Privacy: ✿ ✿ ✿ ✿
Quiet: ✿ ✿ ✿ ✿
Spaciousness: ✿ ✿ ✿ ✿
Security: ✿ ✿ ✿ ✿
Cleanliness: ✿ ✿ ✿ ✿

but was rejected because it lacked a deep-water port. To this day, loads of historical canal structures still stand in and around Williamsport. Jordan Junction hiker/biker site (Mile 101.2) also uses the parking area at Williamsport, 1.4 miles downstream. A word of warning if you're boating in this area: dams above and at Williamsport mean you have to portage on the West Virginia side.

North Mountain hiker/biker site is next, at Mile 110. Parking is 0.4 miles upstream at McCoys Ferry, which is a drive-in campsite (see page 20). The section between this campsite and the previous is nicely wild, with little evidence of human usage, either modern or historical. But just a couple of miles beyond North Mountain hiker/biker site is Fort Frederick, a 250-year-old treasure that is worth a half-day's poking around. (For information on camping at Fort Frederick, see profile on page 42). Then, things start to get rural again.

Next up is Licking Creek hiker/biker site (Mile 116). I wouldn't necessarily recommend it, as it sits very near I-70 and you can hear the traffic at night. In fact, the parking area for this campsite is adjacent to the I-70 exit ramp at Indian Springs (Exit 9), 0.7 miles upstream.

The next four hiker/biker sites all share the same parking area at Little Tonoloway, which has a boat launch, restaurants, groceries, phone, and the visitor center in the town of Hancock. Unfortunately, the first of those four campsites, Little Pool (Mile 120.6), also sits right next to I-70; I wouldn't recommend it either. But if you can stand the noise, the site is 3.9 miles downstream of Little Tonoloway. To reach Little Tonoloway, take Route 522 toward Hancock from I-70 (Exit 3).

The White Rock hiker/biker site (Mile 126.4) inexplicably doesn't show up on some NPS canal literature, but I did confirm that it still exists as of summer 2007. Just a mile upstream is what remains of the Round Top Cement Mill. While the redbrick mill remains only as an intact smokestack and some crumbling walls, the nearby kilns, eight of them total, still look great and are largely intact. By all means check them out, but be aware of the three bat species (big brown, little brown, and Eastern pipistrelle) that hibernate there.

KEY INFORMATION

ADDRESS: C&O Canal NHP Headquarters 1850 Dual Highway, Suite 100 Hagerstown, MD 21740-6620 (301) 739-4200

OPERATED BY: National Park Service

OPEN: All year

SITES: 11

EACH SITE HAS: Grill, chemical toilet, picnic table, and pump well water (but plan for the possibility of a pump not working)

ASSIGNMENT: First come, first served

REGISTRATION: None

FACILITIES: Varies by site; see text

PARKING: Vehicles must be left at the nearest parking area; see text for individual sites

FEE: Free

RESTRICTIONS: *Pets:* None
Quiet Hours: None
Visitors: Max. 8 people per site
Fires: In fire rings or portable grills only
Alcohol: Not allowed
Stay Limit: 1 night per site, per trip
Other: Only dead wood can be collected for fires

MAP

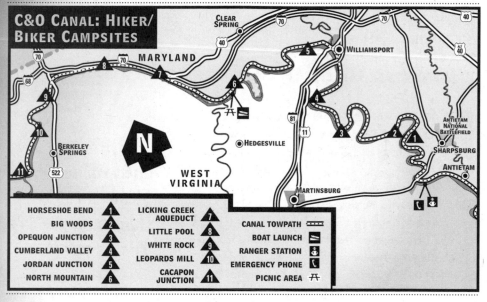

C&O CANAL: HIKER/ BIKER CAMPSITES

HORSESHOE BEND	1	LICKING CREEK AQUEDUCT	7	CANAL TOWPATH	
BIG WOODS	2	LITTLE POOL	8	BOAT LAUNCH	
OPEQUON JUNCTION	3	WHITE ROCK	9	RANGER STATION	
CUMBERLAND VALLEY	4	LEOPARDS MILL	10	EMERGENCY PHONE	
JORDAN JUNCTION	5	CACAPON JUNCTION	11	PICNIC AREA	
NORTH MOUNTAIN	6				

GETTING THERE

Varies; see text.

Leopards Mill hiker/biker site (Mile 129.9) is 5.4 miles upstream of Little Tonoloway, one of the longer hikes to reach a campsite in the C&O Canal system. An even longer hike is the one to Cacapon Junction (Mile 133.6), which is a solid 6.8 miles upstream from Little Tonoloway—no terrible haul if you're on a bike, but a bit of a slog if you've got all your equipment on your back. Cacapon Junction is the area where the Cacapon River, one of my favorite Potomac tributary rivers, meets the Potomac on the West Virginia side.

GPS COORDINATES

UTM Zone (NAD27) 18S
Easting 261606
Northing 4374461

07
C&O CANAL:
HIKER/BIKER CAMPSITES
FROM INDIGO NECK (MILE 139)
TO EVITTS CREEK (MILE 180)

FOR GENERAL INFORMATION on hiker/biker sites, read "C&O Canal: Hiker/Biker Campsites from Swain's Lock (Mile 16.6) to Killiansburg Cave (Mile 75.2)" on page 23. What follows is a continuation of those sites from Cacapon Junction (Mile 133), moving northwesterly along the C&O Canal toward Cumberland.

The first five hiker/biker campsites in this section all sit within or adjacent to the Green Ridge State Forest, which offers fantastic camping opportunities. (For a description of Green Ridge camping, see page 54.) The first site, Indigo Neck (Mile 139.2), uses the parking area 1.6 miles upstream at Fifteen Mile Creek, which is a drive-in site (see page 20). Sideling Hill Creek, a little Potomac tributary that begins in Pennsylvania, is just south of the Indigo Neck hiker/biker site. To get to the parking area at Fifteen Mile Creek, take I-68 and exit at Little Orleans Road (Exit 68).

Devils Alley (Mile 144.5), the next hiker/biker site, also uses the parking area at Fifteen Mile Creek, this time 3.7 miles downstream.

Stickpile Hill (Mile 149.4) and Sorrel Ridge (Mile 154.1) hiker/biker sites are next; as mentioned above, they are all adjacent to the Green Ridge State Forest, which offers a tremendous amount of recreational activity.

After Sorrel Ridge, the towpath breaks up a bit just after Lock 62 as the river squiggles in a series of little bends. To continue hiking upstream, toward Paw Paw Tunnel and Paw Paw drive-in campsite (see page 21), you can take the Tunnel Hill Trail.

Use the Paw Paw campsite parking for both Stickpile Hill and Sorrel Ridge. For Stickpile, Paw Paw is 6.6 miles upstream, and for Sorrel, it's 1.9 miles upstream. To reach Paw Paw, take I-68 to Exit 62 into the Green

> *The first five hiker/ biker campsites in this section all sit within or adjacent to the Green Ridge State Forest.*

RATINGS

Beauty: ✿ ✿ ✿ ✿
Privacy: ✿ ✿ ✿ ✿
Quiet: ✿ ✿ ✿ ✿
Spaciousness: ✿ ✿ ✿ ✿
Security: ✿ ✿ ✿ ✿
Cleanliness: ✿ ✿ ✿ ✿

KEY INFORMATION

ADDRESS: C&O Canal NHP
Headquarters
1850 Dual Highway,
Suite 100
Hagerstown, MD
21740-6620
(301) 739-4200

OPERATED BY: National Park
Service

OPEN: All year

SITES: 10

EACH SITE HAS: Grill, chemical toilet,
picnic table, and
pump well water
(but plan for the
possibility of a pump
not working)

ASSIGNMENT: First come, first
served

REGISTRATION: None

FACILITIES: Varies by site; see
text

PARKING: Vehicles must be left
at the nearest park-
ing area; see text for
individual sites

FEE: Free

RESTRICTIONS: *Pets:* None
Quiet Hours: None
Visitors: Max. 8
people per site
Fires: In fire rings or
portable grills only
Alcohol: Not allowed
Stay Limit: 1 night
per site, per trip
Other: Only dead
wood can be col-
lected for fires

Ridge Forest, on Green Ridge Road West. Head south on Route 51 just before Town Creek Aqueduct.

Purslane Run (Mile 157.4) is next, also using the Paw Paw parking area, this time 1.6 miles downstream. Aside from Green Ridge State Forest, the big attraction here is the Paw Paw Tunnel, by far the most impressive engineering marvel along the canal. Paw Paw Tunnel stretches 3,100 feet and was constructed between 1836 and 1850. The drive-in campsite at Paw Paw gives access to picnic areas, phones, a camp store, and nearby restaurants.

Town Creek Aqueduct (Mile 162.1) is the next hiker/biker campsite, sitting on the westernmost edge of the state forest. Town Creek runs just north of the state forest and empties into the Potomac just north of the campsite. A little north of that, just past Lock 68, the south and north branches of the Potomac meet. To reach the Town Creek hiker/biker site, take I-68 to Exit 62 into the Green Ridge Forest, on Green Ridge Road West. Because the road ends just before the campsite, the camping area can potentially feel a bit crowded. That said, this is not a major traffic thoroughfare.

Where the two branches of the Potomac meet is where you'll find the next hiker/biker site, the aptly named Potomac Forks, at Mile 164.8. I find this to be an especially scenic spot and it's one of my favorite campsites. Just to the north of it looms Warrior Mountain. At 2,185 feet, it's Maryland's seventh highest. Parking for Potomac Forks is 1.9 miles upstream, at Oldtown. To reach it, follow the directions above for Town Creek Aqueduct but head north on Route 51.

Pigmans Ferry hiker/biker site (Mile 169.1) also uses the parking area at Oldtown, this time 1.4 miles downstream. The Spring Gap drive-in site is at Mile 173.3, where you can get take advantage of many amenities; for a full description, see page 21.

Next up is Irons Mountain hiker/biker site (Mile 175.3). For Irons Mountain, use the parking area 2 miles upstream, at North Branch boat launch. Take I-68 to Exit 43C in Cumberland to Route 51 South. This campsite sits near a noisy railroad trestle, so be warned. Perhaps you'd be better off in the next hiker/biker site,

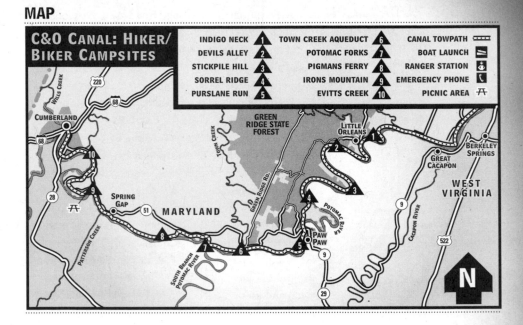

C&O CANAL: HIKER/ BIKER CAMPSITES

INDIGO NECK 1	TOWN CREEK AQUEDUCT 6	CANAL TOWPATH	
DEVILS ALLEY 2	POTOMAC FORKS 7	BOAT LAUNCH	
STICKPILE HILL 3	PIGMANS FERRY 8	RANGER STATION	
SORREL RIDGE 4	IRONS MOUNTAIN 9	EMERGENCY PHONE	
PURSLANE RUN 5	EVITTS CREEK 10	PICNIC AREA	

Evitts Creek (Mile 180.1), the final campsite along the C&O Canal. In fact, heading to Irons Mountain using the directions above will take you past Evitts Creek (though you can't park there). Parking for Evitts Creek is 4.4 miles upstream at the Western Maryland Terminus, the end point for the canal towpath, in the town of Cumberland. There's a visitor center here, as well as bike rentals, groceries, and phone.

Cumberland itself is worth a day of poking around. I especially like the idea of parking here, spending some hours checking things out, and then walking or biking the 4.4 miles to the Evitts Creek campsite. Of course, I wouldn't be the only one with this idea, and it's not unreasonable to expect that the campsite, so close to a large town and the end of a line, may be occupied. The sewage disposal plant at Mile 181.2 is rather unpleasant, but the smell dissipates quickly after leaving the plant behind.

GETTING THERE

Varies; see text.

GPS COORDINATES

UTM Zone (NAD27) 17S
Easting 725739
Northing 4390212

> *The park's namesake is a 78-foot waterfall, which qualifies as Maryland's largest cascading waterfall.*

CUNNINGHAM **FALLS STATE PARK** is situated in the Catoctin Mountains. The park's namesake is a 78-foot waterfall, which qualifies as Maryland's largest cascading waterfall. Franklin Roosevelt first used the area north of Cunningham Falls State Park as a presidential retreat in 1942, trying to escape the oppressive heat of D.C. summers. He named it "Shangri-La." When Roosevelt died, there was some controversy over whether the land would remain in federal hands or revert to Maryland state parkland. A compromise was reached: north of Route 77 would remain under federal control, while land south, today's Cunningham Falls State Park, would go back to Maryland. Today, Cunningham Falls State Park has two separate camping sections: William Houck and Manor.

William Houck is by far the larger of the two campgrounds in the park. This is because it sits next to the park's main attractions: Hunting Creek Lake (with its boating and fishing) and Cunningham Falls. Hunting Creek Lake is a put-and-take trout area, with bass, bluegills, catfish, crappie, and sunfish. Big Hunting Creek, the lake's feeder, provides more fishing opportunities.

Cunningham Falls is an easy half-mile hike from the Houck camping area along the Falls Trail. The park itself has lots of hiking trails, including a mostly isolated one (part of the Catoctin Trail) heading to the Manor camping area. Additionally, the park's fluid border with Catoctin Mountain Park (see page 16) assures even more hiking opportunities nearby.

My favorite trail within the park is Cat Rock/Bob's Hill, which runs 7.5 miles across the mountain and takes in scenic rock outcroppings. It's also easy to link this to Catoctin Mountain Park's trails to more vistas, including Chimney Rock and Wolf Rock. While you're at it, try the Old Misery Trail—if nothing else,

RATINGS

Beauty: ✿ ✿ ✿ ✿ ✿
Privacy: ✿ ✿ ✿
Spaciousness: ✿ ✿ ✿ ✿
Quiet: ✿ ✿ ✿
Security: ✿ ✿ ✿ ✿ ✿
Cleanliness: ✿ ✿ ✿ ✿ ✿

you've got to love the (somewhat misleading) name.

Sites in Cunningham Falls State Park are wooded and large. There is also a camp store near the entrance road next to the Addison Run Loop, which has 25 sites. Addison Run is one of five loops here. The others are Bear Branch (sites 26 to 57), Catoctin Creek (58 to 88), Deer Spring Branch (89 to 117), and Elderberry (118 to 158). Of these, the electric sites are concentrated on the Addison Run Loop (though there are some electric sites in the other loops: Site 44 in Bear Branch, Site 79 in Catoctin Creek, sites 98, 113, 115, and 117 in Deer Spring Branch, and Site 130 in Elderberry). Each loop has its own bathhouse. With all of this activity, your chances for solitude and privacy aren't great, but you can increase them by heading to Elderberry, which is the westernmost loop and farthest from the concentrated electric sites. In Elderberry, I'd recommend sites 118 to 128 as well as 133 to 138. These seem to be the farthest from other sites, and each backs to the woods without any other camping behind. However, the best of the best, if privacy is what you're after, are 102, 104, 105, and 107 in Deer Spring Branch Loop; all of them back up to woods and are very private.

KEY INFORMATION

ADDRESS: **Cunningham Falls State Park**
14039 Catoctin Hollow Road
Thurmont, MD 21788
(301) 271-7574

OPERATED BY: **Maryland Department of Natural Resources**

OPEN: **Addison and Deer Spring Loops, last weekend in April–October; all other loops, Memorial Day–Labor Day**

SITES: **140 (9 camper cabins)**

EACH SITE HAS: **Picnic table, fire ring, lantern post, tent pad**

ASSIGNMENT: **Reservations recommended**

REGISTRATION: **At campground registration off Catoctin Hollow Road, or call (888) 432-CAMP (2267), or online at http://reservations.dnr.state.md.us**

FACILITIES: **Bathhouse, camp store, boat launch, concessions, dump station, playground, water**

PARKING: **In designated camp spots**

FEE: **$25/night, $30/night with electric. Day-use service charge: Memorial Day–Labor Day, $3/person weekdays, $4/person weekends and holidays; all other times, $3/vehicle. Boat launch: $3/vehicle, out-of-state residents add $1 to all service charges**

RESTRICTIONS: *Pets:* **Not permitted**
Quiet Hours: **11 p.m.–7 a.m.**
Visitors: **Must pay per-person fee and be out by 10 p.m.**
Fires: **In fire rings**
Alcohol: **Permitted**
Stay Limit: **2 weeks and can return after 2 weeks**
Other: **Check-out 3 p.m.**

MAP

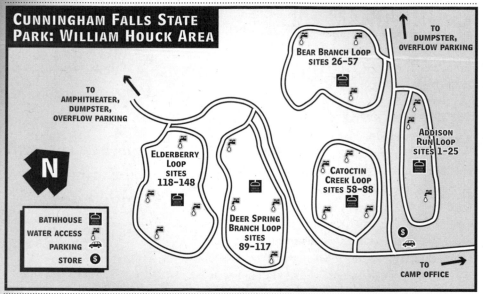

CUNNINGHAM FALLS STATE PARK: WILLIAM HOUCK AREA

TO DUMPSTER, OVERFLOW PARKING

BEAR BRANCH LOOP SITES 26-57

TO AMPHITHEATER, DUMPSTER, OVERFLOW PARKING

ADDISON RUN LOOP SITES 1-25

N

ELDERBERRY LOOP SITES 118-148

CATOCTIN CREEK LOOP SITES 58-88

DEER SPRING BRANCH LOOP SITES 89-117

BATHHOUSE
WATER ACCESS
PARKING
STORE

TO CAMP OFFICE

GETTING THERE

Take I-70 to Frederick, and US 15 North to Thurmont. Follow MD Route 77 West, 4 miles to Catoctin Hollow Road.

If you've brought the kids, don't miss the Catoctin Wildlife Preserve and Zoo, just across Route 15 in Thurmont. With more than 400 animals—from rare monkeys and birds to jaguars, lions, and tigers—it's a great place to spend a few hours.

GPS COORDINATES

UTM Zone (NAD27) 18S
Easting 288278
Northing 4388598

09
CUNNINGHAM FALLS STATE PARK:
MANOR AREA

THE FIRST SETTLERS ARRIVED at the foot of the Catoctin Mountains, in the Monocacy River valley, around 1730. The area's abundance of natural resources assured that industry wouldn't be too far behind. The starkest reminder of that time is the Catoctin Iron Furnace. In use from 1776 until the beginning of the 20th century, the furnace cast raw iron and iron tools. It once churned out ammunition for the Continental Army in the Revolutionary War. One of the brothers who founded the furnace would become governor of Maryland soon after. The furnace ran on charcoal, and the surrounding forests were slowly denuded to provide the requisite fuel. Fortunately, it's been more than a century since the practice stopped, and the area, now Cunningham Falls State Park, has returned once more to an almost pristine state. The furnace is situated very close to the Manor camping area and remains a relatively easy and popular hike from the end of the picnic area. Also nearby (running right through the camping area) is Little Hunting Creek, which provides put-and-take trout fishing.

The Manor Camping Area has are 31 sites total. There are only one-fifth the number of sites of the William Houck Area here, and many people regard the Manor Area as a second choice if they couldn't get a place in William Houck. As a result, unless it's high season and a weekend, you very well may have a good chunk of the camping area to yourself.

Electric sites in the Manor area are 6, 7, 9, 10, 15, and 17 to 21. They are cleverly lined along internal camp roads, which means that the outer sites, away from those internal roads, remain quiet. The most private of these outer sites are 1 to 3, 13, and 23 to 29. From the Manor area, you can easily reach the park's other attractions by taking the Catoctin Trail, a 27-mile trail that runs from south of Frederick in Gambrill

> *The area has returned once more to an almost pristine state.*

RATINGS

Beauty: ✪ ✪ ✪ ✪ ✪
Privacy: ✪ ✪ ✪ ✪
Spaciousness: ✪ ✪ ✪
Quiet: ✪ ✪ ✪ ✪
Security: ✪ ✪ ✪ ✪ ✪
Cleanliness: ✪ ✪ ✪ ✪ ✪

State Park, through Frederick, and into Cunningham Falls State Park; the portion of the trail within the park boundaries runs just under 9 miles. The trail also functions as a popular spur of the Appalachian Trail, which is merely 2 miles away where Raven Rock Road (MD Route 491) and Fort Ritchie Road intersect.

The Manor area sits not far off US 15; by contrast, Houck is several miles within park boundaries. This proximity to US 15 is off-putting to some people, but I've never heard road noise at Manor. The area is sufficiently forested, and US 15 is not a very heavily traveled road, especially at night, so I wouldn't count this proximity as a detraction; however, those seeking complete solitude should at least note the location.

KEY INFORMATION

ADDRESS:	Cunningham Falls State Park
	14039 Catoctin
	Hollow Road
	Thurmont, MD 21788
	(301) 271-7574
OPERATED BY:	Maryland Department of Natural Resources
OPEN:	Family camping season: Memorial Day–August. First come, first served available the first weekend in April–Memorial Day, Labor Day–October, Thanksgiving–mid-December
SITES:	31
EACH SITE HAS:	Dust pad, picnic table, fire ring, lantern post
ASSIGNMENT:	First come, first served April–Memorial Day and Labor Day–end of the season; reservations recommended otherwise
REGISTRATION:	At campground registration off Catoctin Hollow Road, or call (888) 432-CAMP (2267), or online at http://reservations.dnr.state.md.us
FACILITIES:	Bathhouse, playground, picnic area
PARKING:	In designated sites
FEE:	$25/night; $30/night electric. Day-use service charge: Memorial Day–Labor Day, $3/person weekdays; $4/person weekends and holidays; all other times, $3/vehicle
RESTRICTIONS:	*Pets:* Allowed
	Quiet Hours: 11 p.m.–7 a.m.
	Visitors: Must pay per-person fee and be out by 10 p.m.
	Fires: In fire rings
	Alcohol: Permitted
	Stay Limit: 2 weeks, can return after 2 weeks
	Other: Check-out 3 p.m.

MAP

CUNNINGHAM FALLS STATE PARK: MANOR AREA

N

CAMPSITE
BATHHOUSE
WATER ACCESS

GETTING THERE

From Frederick, take US 15
North toward Thurmont.
The Manor area is 3 miles
south of Thurmont
directly off US 15.

GPS COORDINATES

UTM Zone (NAD27) 18S
Easting 290804
Northing 4384641

10
DEEP CREEK LAKE STATE PARK:
MEADOW MOUNTAIN CAMPGROUND

> *Many Marylanders would be surprised to know that this portion of their state actually lies west of the Eastern Continental Divide.*

THE OBVIOUS MAIN ATTRACTION here is the proximity to Deep Creek Lake, a 3,900-acre lake and a four-season recreation area that draws from several surrounding states. Many Marylanders would be surprised to know that this portion of their state actually lies west of the Eastern Continental Divide, meaning that rainfall and snowmelt flow to the Mississippi, not the Atlantic. Additionally, many Marylanders tend to think of water when they think of recreation (the Atlantic and the Chesapeake, of course), which makes Garrett County more popular with those in Pennsylvania and Ohio than many eastern-minded Maryland residents. Deep Creek Lake State Park is the best of both worlds: water and mountains. Abutting both Meadow Mountain and Deep Creek Lake, it offers even more of an attraction: while much of the real estate surrounding the lake has skyrocketed and pushed rental rates beyond the means of many working families, the state park's campgrounds offer a great alternative.

What surrounds the campground is what makes camping here worth it even if you find the site too populated. The vast majority of campers cross over State Park Road to head to the lake, which offers a paradise of boating, swimming, and fishing. Additionally, day-users generally congregate on and near the lake, too.

If you want to escape the crush, it's easy to do so. Don't expect to have the hiking trails all to yourself, but don't expect much traffic either. Deep Creek State Park contains some wonderful trails, all easily accessible from the campground. So while it seems everyone is heading south to the lake, you can go north and escape. (Do leave time for enjoying the lake, however). Had you been hiking here a century ago, virgin red spruce, hemlock, white pine, and yellow birch would have been the dominant tree species, but massive

RATINGS

Beauty: ✿ ✿ ✿ ✿
Privacy: ✿ ✿ ✿
Spaciousness: ✿ ✿ ✿
Quiet: ✿ ✿
Security: ✿ ✿ ✿ ✿ ✿
Cleanliness: ✿ ✿ ✿ ✿ ✿

logging operations cleared the land. Fortunately, the Department of Natural Resources estimates that more than 95 percent of the park has regenerated. Now the forest consists mostly of oak and hickory. Much fauna makes its home here, too, with black bear and bobcat perhaps the most glamorous. The campsites that offer the easiest access to the mountain trails are 34 to 40 in the Delphia Brant Loop and 60 to 67 between the George Beckman and John Garret loops.

Because of its location in such a popular tourist area, Deep Creek State Park doesn't allow for much isolation. (Additionally, the campground is open only during warmer weather months; shoot for April, May, or October for fewer crowds). But for those looking not for a backcountry experience but for a wonderful way to spend some time full of activities, the park is perfect. Its Discover Center offers hands-on exhibits and programs highlighting the area's natural and cultural heritage. Park rangers and naturalists regularly schedule hikes and evening campfire programs that are always fun and informative.

After entering on State Park Road and passing the camp headquarters, you'll immediately come to two loops: one to the left (Meshach Browning Loop) and one to the right (Delphia Brant Loop). Straight ahead is the electric RV loop. Meshach Browning has sites 1 to 26, while Delphia Brant contains sites 27 to 52. Five more sites sit along a spur loop just north of Site 40, which leads to camper cabins and a yurt. The first impression of the campground isn't the best one, especially if it's high season. The initial sites are close together and choc-a-bloc with RVs. But don't despair; keep heading away from these first loops. (If you do wind up in either of these loops, try for Site 40, which sits on a nicely

KEY INFORMATION

ADDRESS:	Deep Creek Lake State Park
	898 State Park Road, Swanton, MD 21561
	(301) 387-5563
OPERATED BY:	Maryland Department of Natural Resources
OPEN:	Late April–mid-October
SITES:	112
EACH SITE HAS:	Grill, picnic table, lantern post, tent pad
ASSIGNMENT:	First come, first served late April–late May and early September–mid-October; reservations otherwise
REGISTRATION:	(888) 432-CAMP (2267) or at http://reservations.dnr.state.md.us
FACILITIES:	Ball fields, bathhouses, boat rental and launch, dumping station, concessions, swimming beach, playgrounds, shelters
PARKING:	2 vehicles at site, off-site for additional vehicles
FEE:	$25/night, $30/night electric. Day-use service charge: Memorial Day–Labor Day, $3/person; out-of-state residents add $1 to service charges
RESTRICTIONS:	*Pets:* In Delphia Brant Loop during off-season
	Quiet Hours: 11 p.m.–7 a.m.
	Visitors: Max. 6 people
	Fires: In fire ring only
	Alcohol: Allowed at camp site but not on beach
	Stay Limit: 2 weeks
	Other: This is bear country; take the proper precautions while camping, never leave food in your tent, and store food in places where a bear can't reach.

MAP

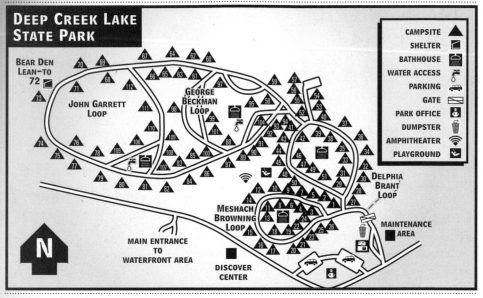

DEEP CREEK LAKE STATE PARK

CAMPSITE
SHELTER
BATHHOUSE
WATER ACCESS
PARKING
GATE
PARK OFFICE
DUMPSTER
AMPHITHEATER
PLAYGROUND

BEAR DEN LEAN-TO 72

JOHN GARRETT LOOP

GEORGE BECKMAN LOOP

DELPHIA BRANT LOOP

MESHACH BROWNING LOOP

MAINTENANCE AREA

N

MAIN ENTRANCE TO WATERFRONT AREA

DISCOVER CENTER

GETTING THERE

Take I-68 to Exit 14A (MD Route 219 South to Deep Creek Lake). Continue on Route 219 South for 18 miles. Turn left onto Glendale Road. Continue on Glendale Road for 1 mile. Immediately after crossing Glendale Bridge, turn left onto State Park Road.

GPS COORDINATES

UTM Zone (NAD27) 17S
Easting 645929
Northing 4375342

wooded corner; to the right of it is the spur loop with sites 52 to 57, dead-end sites with nothing behind them. These aren't bad at all).

Beyond the first loops are the better options: George Beckman and John Garrett Loops, where you'll find sites 58 to 112. Each loop contains its own bathhouse and doesn't differ significantly from the other. But the farther away you go from entrance, the quieter it seems to get and the more spacious the sites. You'll have more privacy here. Site 69 and the sites in the low 70s are nice, sitting on the farthest edge of the campground. My favorite by far is Site 64; it sits behind a big rock ridge and has a trail heading up the hill behind it. The sites in these loops are nice and you should be quite happy with them. I would recommend avoiding only the sites right next to the bathhouse: 81, 95, 97, and 107.

In short, the campsites are reasonably shaded and roomy, each measuring roughly 24 by 24 feet. Still, this is your garden-variety campground—full of basic amenities and with decent tree buffers, but usually crowded. What can't be disputed is that it remains a wonderful alternative to pricier options in this resort area.

11
FORT FREDERICK STATE PARK

FORT **FREDERICK IS PERHAPS** the best place to view the span of Maryland's military history: during the French and Indian War it served as a defense fortification, during the Revolutionary War as a prison, and during the Civil War as a defense of the Chesapeake & Ohio Canal. It proved to be impenetrable, owing to its thick stone walls (at a time when most forts were constructed of wood or earth). Year-round military reenactments, interpretive guides, and a historical center in the fort complex allow for fascinating access to what is considered the country's best-preserved French and Indian stone fort. Restorations begun in the 1920s by the Civilian Conservation Corps have continued all the way through the fort's 250th birthday, celebrated in 2006.

The fort's location makes it a prime attraction. Parkland contains sections of the Potomac River, C&O Canal, Big Pool, and the Western Maryland Rail Trail (WMRT), a 23-mile paved path that follows the former Western Maryland Railway line. The Rails-to-Trails Conservancy recently selected the WMRT as one of the country's best trails for viewing fall foliage. Of course, there's also the C&O Canal Towpath, which follows the Potomac some 185 miles from Washington, D.C., to Cumberland, Maryland. (For camping along the C&O, see pages 19–32).

The Potomac allows for great swimming (be careful: the currents can be deceptively swift midriver), boating, and fishing. The species of fish, both native and introduced, number in the dozens—bass, carp, catfish, crappie, eel, herring, perch, pickerel, shad, sunfish, and trout among them.

One couldn't ask for a better location for a campground. Fort Frederick sits up the hill, easily accessible via a paved path (Fort Frederick Road). Down from

> *The country's best-preserved French and Indian stone fort*

RATINGS

Beauty: ☆ ☆ ☆ ☆
Privacy: ☆ ☆
Spaciousness: ☆ ☆
Quiet: ☆ ☆ ☆ ☆
Security: ☆ ☆ ☆ ☆ ☆
Cleanliness: ☆ ☆ ☆ ☆ ☆

the fort, you cross the C&O Canal Towpath running alongside Big Pool. The campground sits between the towpath and the Potomac River. There are only 29 sites total; 1 to 17 are arguably the best, as they sit waterside (the Potomac), while 18 to 29 sit on the other side of the campground road, nearer Big Pool and the C&O Canal Towpath (not a bad location either). Sites 19 and 20, second- and third-farthest down the campground road, are wheelchair accessible and share a restroom between them. These sites require reservations.

The campground itself is basically one open space, with the sites sitting right next to each other, with 25 feet (and no trees) between them. There's little in the way of privacy. The entire campground is a few hundred yards at best. However, as the sites sit either right alongside the river (1 to 17), or just across the path (18 to 29), there really is no bad spot if you can get over the lack of privacy. The area is very beautiful. One thing to note: there are train tracks on the far side of the river (in West Virginia), so you may hear trains now and again.

KEY INFORMATION

ADDRESS:	Fort Frederick State Park
	11100 Fort Frederick Road
	Big Pool, MD 21711
	(301) 842-2155
OPERATED BY:	Maryland Department of Natural Resources
OPEN:	Early May–late October
SITES:	29
EACH SITE HAS:	Grill, lantern hook, picnic table, tent pad, fire ring
ASSIGNMENT:	Reservations required for wheelchair-accessible sites. Otherwise, you can register at the park or in advance.
REGISTRATION:	(888) 432-CAMP (2267) or at http://reservations.dnr.state.md.us
FACILITIES:	Boat launch, camp store, picnic, playground, shelters, visitor's center
PARKING:	On gravel driveway, max. 2 vehicles per site
FEE:	$15/night; day-use service charge: Memorial Day–Labor Day and weekends in April, May, September, and October, $3/person; tours and special events, year-round $4/person; out-of-state residents add $1 to all day-use charges (service charge applies to historic area only)
RESTRICTIONS:	*Pets:* Allowed on a leash and attended
	Quiet Hours: 11 p.m.–7 a.m.
	Visitors: Max. 6 people
	Fires: In fire rings
	Alcohol: Allowed
	Stay Limit: 2 weeks
	Other: Check-out 3 p.m.

MAP

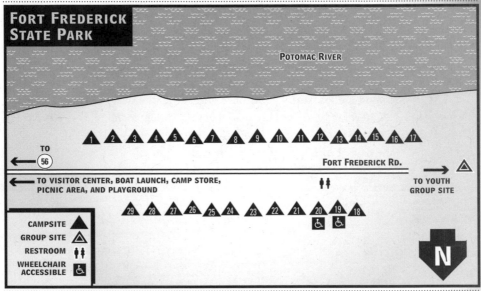

FORT FREDERICK STATE PARK

POTOMAC RIVER

TO 56

1 2 3 4 5 6 7 8 9 10 11 12 13 14 15 16 17

FORT FREDERICK RD.

TO VISITOR CENTER, BOAT LAUNCH, CAMP STORE,
PICNIC AREA, AND PLAYGROUND

TO YOUTH GROUP SITE

29 28 27 26 25 24 23 22 21 20 19 18

CAMPSITE
GROUP SITE
RESTROOM
WHEELCHAIR ACCESSIBLE

N

GETTING THERE

Take I-70 to Exit 12 (Big Pool/Indian Springs, MD Route 56). Turn east on Big Pool Road.

GPS COORDINATES

UTM Zone (NAD27) 17S
Easting 756861
Northing 4388136

> *Because the sites are nicely wooded and relatively minimal in number, the campground rarely feels crowded.*

GAMBRILL STATE PARK, at 1,137 acres, sits within an area of Frederick County that is packed with parks and recreation opportunities. Gambrill sits on a ridge of Catoctin Mountain and contains the summit of High Knob, modest at 1,600 feet but providing some impressive views: Frederick City Municipal Forest to the north, Gathland State Park and the Middletown and Monocacy valleys to the south, and the Civil War historical site, South Mountain, to the west.

Gambrill State Park is divided into two separate recreational areas. Rock Run, at the park entrance, is where you'll find the campground. High Knob encompasses the top of Catoctin Mountain. Midway between the two areas is the Trailhead Parking Lot, which provides access to Gambrill's 16 miles of hiking trails, including access to the Catoctin Trail, a 27-mile trail that traverses Gambrill, Catoctin Mountain Park, Cunningham Falls State Park, and Frederick City Municipal Forest.

The campground at Rock Run sits south of all the trails and is compact and relatively small. This may mean that you're never too far from camping neighbors, but it also means that there will never be too many of them. When I camped here, the place felt relatively empty, though there didn't seem to be too many vacant sites. It's often this way, I was told. Because the sites are nicely wooded and relatively minimal in number, the campground rarely feels crowded. The pace is relaxed. There's also a small pond in Rock Run, stocked with bass, bluegill, and catfish.

There are 34 sites in all, including four full-service cabins numbered 4, 5, 6, and 18. After the electric sites (1, 12, 13, 20, 22), a relatively small number of sites are left for tent campers. Of these, only sites 23 to 27 and 30 to 34 are tent-only. If you want one of these sites,

RATINGS

Beauty: ✪ ✪ ✪ ✪
Privacy: ✪ ✪ ✪
Spaciousness: ✪ ✪
Quiet: ✪ ✪ ✪
Security: ✪ ✪ ✪ ✪ ✪
Cleanliness: ✪ ✪ ✪ ✪

definitely go for 30 to 34. They sit on the farthest section from the entrance, up the hill. In general, the higher up the hill you go, the nicer the sites are. The sites in the first tent-only area, 23 to 27, are in a middle section with roads nearby and very close to one another. Another bonus to the upper sites (30 to 34) is that they sit right in front of the red trail, which you'd take to access all the other park trails. Of these sites, I like the rocks and mature trees that decorate Site 31.

Of course, you're not limited to the tent-only sites, even if you have only a tent. The rule of thumb, again, is to keep heading away from the entrance. The farther you go, the better the sites are. This means that the first ones you come to, 1 to 7 and 19 to 27, are best avoided. Heading away from the entrance, sites 8 to 18 and 30 to 34 are your best bets.

KEY INFORMATION

ADDRESS:	Gambrill State Park
	c/o Cunningham Falls State Park
	14039 Catoctin Hollow Road
	Thurmont, MD 21702
	(301) 271-7574
OPERATED BY:	Maryland Department of Natural Resources
OPEN:	Late April–late October
SITES:	30 (plus 4 camper cabins)
EACH SITE HAS:	Grill, lantern hook, picnic table, tent pad
ASSIGNMENT:	First come, first served May and September–end of the season; reservations always available
REGISTRATION:	For self-registration, pick available site and register within 30 minutes. For reservations, call (888) 432-CAMP (2267) or go to http://reservations.dnr.state.md.us
FACILITIES:	Bathhouses, picnic shelters, playground
PARKING:	All vehicles must be on gravel drive, except in tent-only sites
FEE:	$20/night, $25/night electric, $27/night full hook-up. If over 62 years old and it's Sunday–Thursday, $10/night, $15/night electric, $17/night full hookup. Day-use fee: $3/vehicle, $4/vehicle out-of-state residents
RESTRICTIONS:	*Pets:* On a leash and attended
	Quiet Hours: 11 p.m.–7 a.m.
	Visitors: Max. 8 people per site
	Fires: In fire ring
	Alcohol: Permitted
	Stay Limit: 2 weeks
	Other: Check-out 3 p.m.

MAP

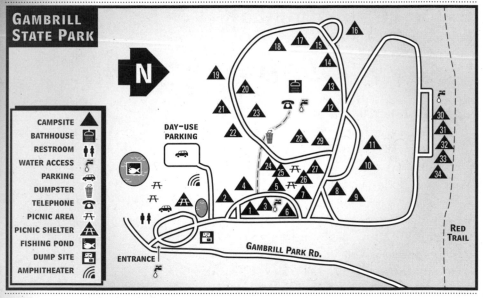

GAMBRILL STATE PARK

N

Legend	
CAMPSITE	▲
BATHHOUSE	🚿
RESTROOM	👥
WATER ACCESS	🚰
PARKING	🚗
DUMPSTER	🗑
TELEPHONE	☎
PICNIC AREA	🪑
PICNIC SHELTER	⛺
FISHING POND	🎣
DUMP SITE	♿
AMPHITHEATER	📡

DAY-USE PARKING

ENTRANCE

GAMBRILL PARK RD.

RED TRAIL

GETTING THERE

Take I-270 or I-70 to Frederick and follow to US Route 15 and then to Route 40 West (pass US Alt. 40) exit to Gambrill Park Road.

GPS COORDINATES

UTM Zone (NAD27) 18S
Easting 285336
Northing 4370715

13

GARRETT STATE FOREST:
SNAGGY MOUNTAIN AREA

A WORD OF WARNING: the Garrett State Forest's camping areas aren't very easy to locate because they're sandwiched between two prominent state parks: Swallow Falls and Herrington Manor. In fact, it's more accurate to say that the two state parks are located within the forest, and the forest is easily mistaken as a greenbelt between Swallow Falls and Herrington Manor. Both state parks have well-established camping facilities (Herrington Manor is cabin-only), and, as a result, people are often unaware that they can camp in the forest as well. The largest and best-maintained camping section in the forest sits between the two parks and is called the Snaggy Mountain Area. It's a wonderful-if-underutilized primitive camping area.

The Garrett State Forest is where forestry conservation in Maryland began. The Garrett Brothers owned the western forestlands in this area, and in 1906 they donated more than 1,900 acres to the state. Today, the holdings that constitute the state forest total more than 7,000 acres. It's an area of rugged and wooded mountain terrain, speckled with streams and rivers and home to an abundance of wildlife.

The camping area sits just off the unpaved Snaggy Mountain Road (see directions below). Taking in portions of Snaggy Mountain Road is the Garrett Trail, a 7-mile hike that offers stunning sights in the forest: river valleys, hemlock groves, and wetlands. The trail also passes (and sometimes encompasses) two other prominent trails: Backbone Mountain and Potomac River. Additionally, a 5.5-mile trail runs through the area and connects the two state parks. At Herrington Manor, a 53-acre lake anchors a popular recreation area. (For a description of Swallow Falls, see page 94).

In short, there's a plethora of hiking opportunities in the Snaggy Mountain Area, all of them within a

> *The sites are all spacious, private, and located in a stunning natural setting.*

RATINGS

Beauty: ✩ ✩ ✩ ✩ ✩
Privacy: ✩ ✩ ✩ ✩ ✩
Quiet: ✩ ✩ ✩ ✩
Spaciousness: ✩ ✩ ✩ ✩ ✩
Security: ✩ ✩ ✩
Cleanliness: ✩ ✩ ✩ ✩ ✩

KEY INFORMATION

ADDRESS: Potomac-Garrett
State Forest
222 Herrington Lane
Oakland, MD 21550
(301) 334-2038

OPERATED BY: Maryland Department of Natural Resources

OPEN: All year, but roads are not maintained in winter

SITES: 11

EACH SITE HAS: Lantern hook, grill, picnic table

ASSIGNMENT: First come, first served

REGISTRATION: Self-registration station on Snaggy Mountain Road

FACILITIES: None

PARKING: Vehicles must be parked on gravel portion of site

FEE: $10/night

RESTRICTIONS: *Pets:* Permitted
Quiet Hours: 11 p.m.–7 a.m.
Visitors: Max. 8 people or 2 units
Fires: In fire rings only
Alcohol: Permitted
Stay Limit: 2 weeks
Other: Check-out is 3 p.m. This is bear country—take proper precautions. For tips on how to camp amongst bears, visit www.dnr.state.md.us /wildlife/bbmd.html

short jaunt from the campsites. Be aware, however, that most forest trails are open not only to hikers but to skiers, equestrians, snowmobilers, and off-road vehicle operators. (The exception to this is the Herrington Manor's Swallow Falls Trail, which doesn't allow motorized vehicles.) Still, don't let this dissuade you from camping here; it's truly a beautiful spot. I would recommend, however, getting hold of a trail map from the Garrett State Forest headquarters (see below for contact info) before setting out. Once you've reached Snaggy Mountain Road from Cranesville Road, the self-registration station is just up ahead. Similar to the Potomac State Forest, which is maintained by the same section of the Department of Natural Resources, the sites are all spacious, private, and located in a stunning natural setting. They also often sit a quarter of a mile or more from one another. And, just like in the Potomac State Forest, you can't go wrong with any one of them. In fact, I would be inclined to simply take the first available site (if nothing else, it saves the jarring on your car). Site 2 is one of the most gorgeous camping spots I've seen. Covered in pine needles, it sits in a grove of hemlocks and has much level ground for tents. You'll see a yellow marked trail to the left just down the road heading toward Site 3.

Because all 11 sites sit along Snaggy Mountain Road, and the road itself has an outlet on both ends (Cranesville to the north and Herrington Manor to the south), the issue of passing cars shouldn't really be part of your equation when picking a site. In any case, passing vehicles will be moving slowly, as the roads are unpaved and very bumpy. Again, simply choose the first available site; you can't go wrong.

MAP

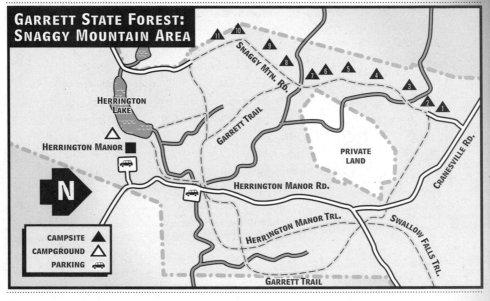

GARRETT STATE FOREST: SNAGGY MOUNTAIN AREA

SNAGGY MTN. RD.

GARRETT TRAIL

HERRINGTON LAKE

HERRINGTON MANOR

PRIVATE LAND

CRANESVILLE RD.

N

HERRINGTON MANOR RD.

HERRINGTON MANOR TRL.

SWALLOW FALLS TRL.

GARRETT TRAIL

CAMPSITE
CAMPGROUND
PARKING

GETTING THERE

From Deep Creek Lake, take MD Route 219 South for 2 miles to a right on Mayhew Inn Road and go 4.5 miles to a stop sign. Turn left onto Oakland Sang Run Road to the first right onto Swallow Falls Road. Pass Swallow Falls State Park and take a right (almost a U-turn) onto Cranesville Road, and then a left onto Snaggy Mountain Road.

GPS COORDINATES

UTM Zone (NAD27) 17S
Easting 635739
Northing 4373270

14
GARRETT STATE FOREST:
PINEY MOUNTAIN AREA AND BACKCOUNTRY CAMPING

> *Camping here is a real out-of-the-way experience, and well worth the trouble locating it.*

I N THE DESCRIPTION OF Garrett State Forest: Snaggy Mountain Area on page 48, I mention that the forest camping area can be difficult to locate. In the case of the Piney Mountain Area of the forest, that goes double. It seems easy enough, but the northern portion of the state forest (where the Piney Mountain Area is located) is a patchwork on non-contiguous public lands surrounded by private holdings. Further, because of the rural nature of the area, there are few markers to guide you.

However, the problems listed above are a byproduct of the fact that camping here is a real out-of-the-way experience, and well worth the necessary trouble locating it. The six sites within the Piney Mountain Area constitute huge, cleared areas carved from the forest that sit along the unpaved Piney Mountain Road. They are essentially identical to the sites in the Snaggy Mountain Area. The real difference between the two is that Piney Mountain is more remote, and doesn't see nearly the same amount of through traffic created by Snaggy Mountain's much closer proximity to Herrington Manor and Swallow Falls State Parks. Also, camping at Piney Mountain offers easy access to one of Maryland's natural oddities. Straddling the Maryland–West Virginia border on Cranesville Road just to the west of the Piney Mountain Area is the Cranesville Swamp. This is a sub-artic swamp, hosting a landscape that one rarely ever finds south of Canada. A perfect storm of environmental conditions created it, and it hosts birds and flowers that otherwise can't be seen this far south.

Piney Mountain Road is an unpaved forest road and leads to a secondary loop trail that disallows motorized vehicles. The campsites sit along the road and are hardly distinguishable from one another—in a good way. They are all spacious, and far from the next

RATINGS

Beauty ✩ ✩ ✩ ✩ ✩
Privacy ✩ ✩ ✩ ✩ ✩
Quiet ✩ ✩ ✩ ✩ ✩
Spaciousness ✩ ✩ ✩ ✩ ✩
Security ✩ ✩ ✩
Cleanliness ✩ ✩ ✩ ✩ ✩

site, and they sit within pristine forest. Like the other sites in Garrett Forest (and Potomac State Forest), you can't go wrong with any one of them. Take the first one that is available; you'll be quite happy with it. Aside from the privacy and out-of-the-way feel of the campsites in Piney Mountain, its general proximity to the two state parks listed above means it's a less expensive, more private alternative, albeit without the facilities one would enjoy at a state park.

If the idea of a fire grill, lantern hook, and picnic table means that in your view, you're not at all roughing it, you can also camp anywhere in the forest where there are not established sites, provided you have obtained a backcountry permit. For Piney Mountain, this effectively means the area south of Sang Run Road and between Piney Mountain Road and Cranesville Road. For the Snaggy Mountain Area (see page 48), this backcountry experience can be had in the large swath of forest between Herrington Manor and Swallow Falls, with the exception of a large privately held area, which is marked accordingly.

KEY INFORMATION

ADDRESS:	Potomac-Garrett State Forest
	222 Herrington Lane
	Oakland, MD 21550
	(301) 334-2038
OPERATED BY:	Maryland Department of Natural Resources
OPEN:	All year (but roads are not maintained in winter)
SITES:	6+ (6 in Piney Mountain Area, unlimited in forest backcountry)
EACH SITE HAS:	Lantern hook, grill, picnic table (Piney Mountain Area)
ASSIGNMENT:	First come, first served
REGISTRATION:	Self-registration station on Piney Mountain Road
FACILITIES:	None
PARKING:	Vehicles must be parked on gravel portion of site, off road in forest
FEE:	$10/night
RESTRICTIONS:	*Pets:* Permitted
	Quiet Hours: 11 a.m.–7 p.m.
	Visitors: 8 people or 2 units max.
	Fires: In fire rings only
	Alcohol: Permitted
	Stay Limit: 2 weeks
	Other: Check-in and check-out is 3 p.m. for roadside sites. Camping is prohibited within 200 feet of any trail or stream. This is bear country; take proper precautions—for tips on how to camp amongst bears, visit: www.dnr.state.md.us/wildlife/bbmd.html

MAP

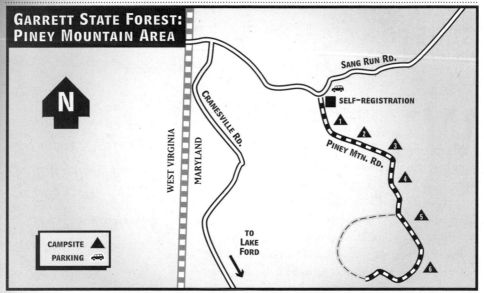

GARRETT STATE FOREST: PINEY MOUNTAIN AREA

N

WEST VIRGINIA

MARYLAND

CRANESVILLE RD.

SANG RUN RD.

SELF-REGISTRATION

PINEY MTN. RD.

TO LAKE FORD

CAMPSITE ▲
PARKING 🚐

GETTING THERE

From I-68, take Exit 14 (MD Route 219 south) for roughly 15 miles to a right on Sang Run Road. Follow to a left onto Piney Mountain Road (if you reach Cranesville Road, turn around and look for Piney Mountain to the right).

GPS COORDINATES

UTM Zone (NAD27) 17S
Easting 632208
Northing 4378921

WANT TO GET AWAY FROM IT ALL? Camping in Green Ridge State Forest is almost too good to be true: 100 widely disbursed primitive and semi-primitive campsites within 44,000 acres of oak and hickory forest.

After Savage River State Forest, Green Ridge is Maryland's second-largest state forest, at 44,000 acres. The forest encompasses Green Ridge Mountain and Polish Mountain, as well as 2,039-foot Town Hill, the forest's highest point. It also happens to be, for what it's worth, my favorite camping destination in Maryland. This is because it's only two hours from my home in Baltimore, lacks the massive crowds heading east to the ocean and the better-known recreation areas to the west, and allows for truly spectacular, away-from-it-all camping. At $10 a night, it's also an absolute bargain.

I've broken up the campsites for Green Ridge State Forest into three entries in this book. Aside from the fact that the unpaved roads and immensity of the forest can make getting from campsite to campsite a long and arduous process, breaking the sites up the way I have done (north of I-68 [sites 1 to 23], east of Green Ridge [53 to 100] and west of Green Ridge [24 to 52]) means that you can choose your campsite based upon one of three options: if you desire a quick and easy escape, go for the sites north of I-68; if you want forested bliss and access to the western hiking trails, go for the west side of Green Ridge; and if you desire forest but wish for easier access to the C&O Canal and the Potomac River, go for the east side of Green Ridge. If you want to choose your stay based on certain activities, here's a rough guide: use sites 1 to 54 for hunting; 24 to 49, 55 to 79, and 86 to 88 for equestrian use; 80 to 85 and 90 to 100 for boating and fishing. No site is terribly far from a hiking trail, and forest roads

> *These are wonderful campsites, all far from one another, all within pristine forested settings, and all with plenty of space to pitch several tents.*

RATINGS

Beauty: ✩ ✩ ✩ ✩ ✩
Privacy: ✩ ✩ ✩ ✩ ✩
Spaciousness: ✩ ✩ ✩ ✩
Quiet: ✩ ✩ ✩ ✩ ✩
Security: ✩ ✩ ✩
Cleanliness: ✩ ✩ ✩ ✩ ✩

KEY INFORMATION

ADDRESS: Green Ridge State Forest
28700 Headquarters Drive, NE
Flintstone, MD 21530-9525
(301) 478-3124

OPERATED BY: Maryland Department of Natural Resources

OPEN: All year

SITES: 23 (100 total in forest)

EACH SITE HAS: Fire ring, picnic table

ASSIGNMENT: First come, first served

REGISTRATION: Campers must register at the Green Ridge Visitor Center (see directions). Use self-registration if the center is closed.

FACILITIES: Bathrooms, water at visitor center

PARKING: On gravel pad, off forest road

FEE: $10/night for up to 6 people, $1 each additional person

RESTRICTIONS: *Pets:* Permitted on a leash
Quiet Hours: None posted
Visitors: See "Fee"
Fires: Permitted at sites but must be monitored at all times
Alcohol: Permitted
Stay Limit: None; when you register, mark the intended length of stay
Other: Individuals registering for the site must be at least 18 years of age.

are, in essence, "hikable" traverses.

Because the campsites are spread out across the forest, a good map is essential. But here's a rough guide for the sites north of I-68: Sites 1 to 23 sit nestled within the following approximate boundaries: I-68 to the south, Fifteen Mile Creek (and Fifteen Mile Creek Road) to the east, Old Cumberland Road to the north, and Treasure Road and Frank Davis Road to the west. It's evident that you'll be near a road no matter what. But these are narrow, unpaved forest roads that don't see much traffic. It is reasonable, however, to want to be far away from I-68, which sees trucks throughout the night. However, you might be surprised by how quiet this area is despite its proximity to the interstate. The only two sites where you might hear road noise are those closest: Site 1 on Fifteen Mile Creek Road and Site 19 on Big Ridge Road. Site 1 is certainly the most convenient and will spare you the jarring of the roads, but my suggestion is to continue north along Fifteen Mile Creek Road and take the next left onto Carpenter Road. The first site you'll come to, on the right, is Site 11. This is a fantastic site, large and deep in the woods. Plus, you can easily walk back to Fifteen Mile and pick up the red trail just behind. It is labeled the Pine Lick Trail, and its terminus at the Mason-Dixon Line links with the 176-mile Mid-State Pennsylvania Trail.

Sites 12 to 15 are found continuing west along Carpenter. (If you have a large group, take Site 12, it's enormous.) Sites 2 to 4 are north up Fifteen Mile Creek Road. Just beyond Carpenter Road north is Double Pine Road, where you'll find sites 5 to 10, as well as a shelter site, convenient in case of bad weather. This site is off the little path just south of Site 10. The rest in this section: use Old Cumberland Road for Site 4 (left from Fifteen Mile). Use Davis Road for sites 20 to 22 (left off Carpenter after the intersection with Treasure Road, which you would use to get to Site 23, one of the most remote sites in all the forest). Last, use Big Ridge Road for sites 16 to 19 (the second left off Fifteen Mile just after exiting I-68).

All of these sites sit right off the forest road, so they're easy to find. However, using a good map is

MAP

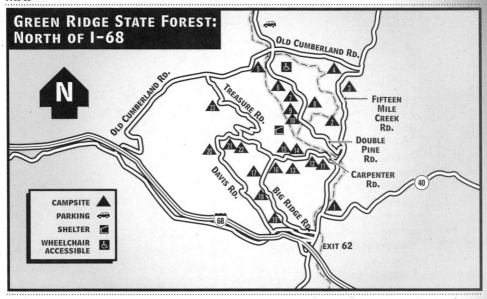

GREEN RIDGE STATE FOREST: NORTH OF I-68

OLD CUMBERLAND RD.

OLD CUMBERLAND RD.

TREASURE RD.

FIFTEEN MILE CREEK RD.

DOUBLE PINE RD.

CARPENTER RD.

DAVIS RD.

BIG RIDGE RD.

EXIT 62

40

68

CAMPSITE
PARKING
SHELTER
WHEELCHAIR ACCESSIBLE

essential. That said, the relentless pitch and yaw of your car on these roads means you'll probably want to simply find a suitable site and stop. Using the directions to the right as a rough guide, just go until you find a site that's perfect for you; you won't have to go far. When you find the one you want, you can call the visitor center (where you need to stop first and pay) and tell them where you are. These are wonderful campsites, all far from one another, all within pristine forested settings, and all with plenty of space to pitch several tents.

GETTING THERE

To the visitor center: Take I-68 Exit 64 south (M.V. Smith Road) to right at the visitor center. Once registered, go back to I-68 West to Exit 62, Fifteen Mile Creek Road North.

GPS COORDINATES

UTM Zone (NAD27) 17S
Easting 717538
Northing 4397513

> *This region sees the lowest annual precipitation in the state ... be on the lookout for prickly pear cactus.*

LIKE MUCH OF WESTERN MARYLAND'S forest-land, Green Ridge was once denuded of trees. Beginning in the early 1800s, business ventures gave it a go in the land that now comprises the forest. Almost unbelievably, the entire area was cleared in hopes of turning it into "the largest apple orchard in the universe." That enterprise failed. But the damage had been done. That reality precludes a walk within soaring, centuries-old growth. However, the forest has regenerated and now stands at some 70 years in places.

This forest is best enjoyed west of Green Ridge, in the rising valley lands between Town Hill to the east and Polish Mountain to the west. Aside from some great hiking, there's also the forest's prime designated mountain-bike trail, 12 miles of up and down through some stunning scenery. It seems that most of my camping trips are saturated with rainfall. If that's your experience too, Green Ridge may be a good place to hedge your bets. This region sees the lowest annual precipitation in the state. A bizarre result of this: be on the lookout for prickly pear cactus as you're hiking (yes, you read that correctly!).

Sites 24 through 52 lie southwest of I-68 and west of Green Ridge, the natural dividing line in the forest. Again, each site sits just off a forest road, so consult a good map. As pointed out in the previous entry in this book, there really isn't a bad site in the Green Ridge State Forest; my recommendation is to simply drive past them until you either tire of the bouncing road or find one that suits your needs. Chances are, you won't have to travel too far. What you hope to focus on during your stay will determine where you'll want to pitch your tent: most of the activity in this section is centered near Wallizer Road, where there's mountain-bike trail parking, horseback riding, and fishing at White Sulphur Pond. Sites 29 to 32, as well as a group site

RATINGS

Beauty: ✿ ✿ ✿ ✿ ✿
Privacy: ✿ ✿ ✿ ✿ ✿
Spaciousness: ✿ ✿ ✿ ✿ ✿
Quiet: ✿ ✿ ✿ ✿ ✿
Security: ✿ ✿ ✿
Cleanliness: ✿ ✿ ✿ ✿ ✿

(G1), sit near the pond along Wallizer. The main artery in this section is Green Ridge Road, which runs perpendicular to Wallizer. Sites 33 and 34 are also accessed using Green Ridge Road. Use Sugar Bottom Road for sites 24 to 28—these sites are also near the activities listed above but are not as close as those on Wallizer. If you prefer to stay far away from the action, head west, using Jacobs Road, for sites 41 and 49; Twigg Road for sites 38 to 40 and 44 to 48; May Road for 42 and 43; Gordon Road for 36 and 37; and Mertens Avenue for 35 and 38 to 40. Be aware that Site 35 on Mertens Avenue sits just across the road from a group site (G2) but is also within easy walking distance of a great overlook south on Green Ridge Road.

Heading south along Fifteen Mile Creek Road from I-68, your second right is Sugar Bottom Road. Fifteen Mile then begins to zigzag before straightening out at Green Ridge Road (you have to veer right to get onto Green Ridge; if you pass Site 55 to the left, you've gone too far). Now on Green Ridge, Wallizer is your next right; sites G1 and 32 are the first you come to, each close to White Sulphur Pond; sites 33 and 34 are next along Green Ridge; then Mertens Avenue appears on the right. The first right off Mertens is Gordon Road (36 and 37, closest to the bike trails). Where you would turn right for Gordon, going left instead takes you past sites 38 to 40 and then to Twigg Road (left, sites 44 to 48) and May Road (right, Site 42), and finally Jacobs Road (head right for Site 41, left for 49 to 52). Be aware that these last three sites are quite far, requiring a real bumpy ride. An easier way to access sites 50 to 52 is by continuing on Green Ridge South and taking a right on Jacobs. Doing this will also take you past the fantastic Warrior Mountain Overlook, named for The Great Warrior Path, a Native American trail linking the Carolinas to the Great Lakes.

MAP

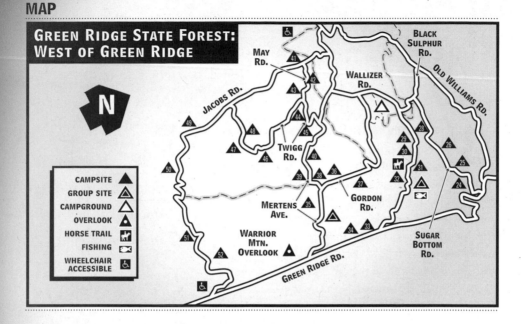

GREEN RIDGE STATE FOREST: WEST OF GREEN RIDGE

N

CAMPSITE ▲
GROUP SITE ⛤
CAMPGROUND △
OVERLOOK ⛰
HORSE TRAIL 🏇
FISHING 🎣
WHEELCHAIR ACCESSIBLE ♿

GETTING THERE

To visitor center: Take I-68 Exit 64 south (M.V. Smith Road) to right at center. Once registered, go back to I-68 West to Exit 62, Fifteen Mile Creek Road South.

GPS COORDINATES

UTM Zone (NAD27) 17S
Easting 717310
Northing 4393517

17
GREEN RIDGE
STATE FOREST:
EAST OF GREEN RIDGE

AS INDICATED IN THE PREVIOUS ENTRIES in this book, Green Ridge State Forest is steeped in history. Unfortunately, early enterprises denuded the area. From landowners such as George Washington to relatives of the Constitution's signers, many folks had a hand in "taming" the landscape. But the forest has grown back to great effect. (The history hasn't disappeared, however; to this day, a drive down Old Town Road follows the route originally cut in the 1750s to link Fort Frederick in the south to Fort Cumberland in the north.)

This section of the forest is characterized by its drop (losing about 700-plus feet of altitude) as it heads toward the Potomac River; here you'll find Green Ridge State Forest's most well-maintained infrastructure. Assuming you're heading south along Green Ridge Road from the I-68 exit at Fifteen Mile Creek Road, you'll first pass the left turn to sites 55 and 56 just after the road stops its switchbacks. It's then a long ride (more than 2 miles) to a left on Mertens Road, heading east. You'll first come to sites 53 and 54. You might very well be tired of the jarring at this point, but I'd recommend you keep going (more on why in a moment). Continuing east on Mertens, you'll first cross Stafford Road (home of sites 57 to 63, which you'll reach in descending numerical order if you go north). If you go right down Stafford, you'll come to Site 100, which sits by itself where Stafford and East Valley Road meet, not far from fishing at Orchard Pond. I would recommend very strongly that you skip all of these sites, as they sit on or very near the ORV trails, which constitute a large loop from Stafford to East Valley Road. Off-roading here is prominently advertised, and I wouldn't risk the noise.

If you keep heading east on Mertens, you'll pass group site G7, and next up is Oldtown Orleans Road,

> *A drive down Old Town Road follows the route originally cut in the 1750s.*

RATINGS

Beauty: ✰ ✰ ✰ ✰ ✰
Privacy: ✰ ✰ ✰ ✰ ✰
Spaciousness: ✰ ✰ ✰ ✰
Quiet: ✰ ✰ ✰ ✰ ✰
Security: ✰ ✰ ✰
Cleanliness: ✰ ✰ ✰ ✰ ✰

KEY INFORMATION

ADDRESS: Green Ridge
State Forest
28700 Headquarters
Drive NE
Flintstone, MD
21530-9525
(301) 478-3124

OPERATED BY: Maryland Department of Natural
Resources

OPEN: All year

SITES: 48, plus 5 group sites
(100 total in forest)

EACH SITE HAS: Fire ring, picnic
table

ASSIGNMENT: First come, first
served

REGISTRATION: Campers must
register at the Green
Ridge Visitor Center
(see directions). Use
self-registration if
the center is closed.

FACILITIES: Bathrooms, water at
visitor center

PARKING: On gravel pad, off
forest road

FEE: $10/night for up to
6 people, $1 each
additional person

RESTRICTIONS: *Pets:* Permitted on a
leash
Quiet Hours: None
posted
Visitors: See "Fee"
Fires: Permitted at
sites but must be
monitored at all
times
Alcohol: Permitted
Stay Limit: None;
when you register,
mark the intended
length of stay
Other: Individuals
registering for the
site must be at least
18 years of age.

containing Site 64 just to the south and 67 to 69 to the north, as well as group site G4. If you were to continue on Mertens, you'll come to some of my favorites sites, 65 and 66, which you'd reach by going right on Outdoor Club Road. This is a dead end, so it will see no though traffic, and these are the only two sites along its route. It would have taken you a while to get there, but now you can relax on a great site. They sit atop the C&O Canal just in front of a beautiful sweep of the Potomac River, easily accessed.

Had you not continued on Mertens but instead kept heading north on Oldtown Orleans, past G4 and 67 to 69, you'd eventually hit sites 70 to 79. After site 79, you'd find yourself looping back toward sites 57 to 55 and Green Ridge Road, not far from where you came off of I-68. Of these sites, I'd recommend Site 74, which sits completely by itself on Howard Road, a right turn off Oldtown Orleans. (Of course, if you want to take this site initially, take the northern route described above, as opposed to making the enormous loop down Mertens— again, get a detailed map.) After Site 70 on Oldtown Orleans Road, heading south there's a left you can take to reach Carroll Road. By going right on Carroll, you'll find sites 86 to 89, as well as G6 (between 87 and 88).

For the rest of the sites in this section, I'd recommend exiting I-68 at Exit 68 (Orleans Road south). If you do that, in about 3 miles you'll come to Mountain Road. Here you'll find group site G5, plus 80 to 83 by going right on Mountain. Of these, I like 80 and 81 best, as they sit astride Fifteen Mile Creek. If you'd taken a left on Yonkers Bottom Road between G5 and site 83, you'd reach Site 84, a great remote spot on Fifteen Mile Creek. Site 85 is difficult to get to and may not be worth the effort if you go there and it's already taken, but it's an incredible site, completely on its own off Cliff Road above Sideling Hill Creek. (When you go to the visitor center, they can tell you which sites are already occupied.) To reach it, take the second left off Orleans Road (Price Road) and then a right on Hoop Pole Road to a right on Stottlemeyer Road. Look for it on the right.

Lastly, sites 90 to 99 should be your preference if you've brought the canoe or kayak, as they all lie near

MAP

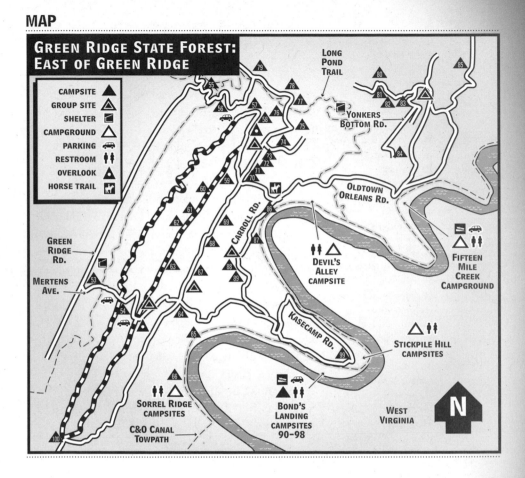

**GREEN RIDGE STATE FOREST:
EAST OF GREEN RIDGE**

CAMPSITE ▲
GROUP SITE △
SHELTER ▣
CAMPGROUND △
PARKING 🚐
RESTROOM 👫
OVERLOOK △
HORSE TRAIL 🏇

LONG POND TRAIL

YONKERS BOTTOM RD.

OLDTOWN ORLEANS RD.

GREEN RIDGE RD.

MERTENS AVE.

CARROLL RD.

KASECAMP RD.

DEVIL'S ALLEY CAMPSITE

FIFTEEN MILE CREEK CAMPGROUND

STICKPILE HILL CAMPSITES

SORREL RIDGE CAMPSITES

C&O CANAL TOWPATH

BOND'S LANDING CAMPSITES 90–98

WEST VIRGINIA

N

---

the Bonds Landing boat launch on Kasecamp Road. Sites 90 to 98 are the few sites in the forest that don't offer too much privacy. You might want to consider Site 99, which offers the best bet for privacy, sitting by itself to the northeast along Kasecamp. You'd reach these sites by going as far east as you can on Mertens and then taking a U-turn right on Kasecamp. (Be aware: this is not an easy trip in any vehicle, and probably not worth the effort if you're trailing a big boat.)

GPS COORDINATES

UTM Zone (NAD27) 17S
Easting 718196
Northing 4387663

GETTING THERE

To visitor center: Take I-68 Exit 64 South (M.V. Smith Road) to right at center. Once registered, go back to I-68 West to Exit 62, Fifteen Mile Creek Road South, for the campsites near Green Ridge. For campsites closer to the C&O Canal and the Potomac, take I-68, Exit 68, Little Orleans Road South.

" *Annapolis Rock has a well-deserved reputation as a place to while away hours simply sitting and taking it all in.* "

GREENBRIER STATE PARK, at just under 1,300 acres, has two main attractions: the Appalachian Trail and the 42-acre Greenbrier Lake. The lake provides good fishing, as it's stocked with trout, largemouth bass, and bluegill. It also serves as a great place for a swim, with its nice beach.

In 2003, the Maryland Conservation Corps and the Potomac Appalachian Trail Club constructed the Bartman's Hill Trail, which leaves from the visitor center and heads directly to the Appalachian Trail. While some 12 miles of trails run throughout the western reaches of the park, many people ignore them and give in to the cache of hiking the AT, even if just for a day or two. Once you reach the AT from the Bartman's Hill Trail, it's 3 miles in either direction to two popular sites: Annapolis Rock to the north and Washington Monument State Park to the south.

At 1,700 feet elevation, Annapolis Rock is fairly modest in height (even by Maryland standards), but the view it commands over Greenbrier Lake and the Cumberland Valley earns it a well-deserved reputation as a place to while away hours simply sitting and taking it all in.

Heading the other way, Washington Monument State Park is a small park at only 108 acres, but it contains a true piece of American history: the country's first monument to our first president. Within a couple of hours, you can see the most famous Washington Monument in D.C. and the most beautiful one in Mount Vernon, Baltimore, but the one that stands in Washington Monument State Park is perhaps the best, for a simple reason: its incredible austerity bestows upon it a singular purity. It stands only 34 feet tall as a circular wall of dry rock.

As for the camping, there are four loops, each with a bathhouse. It's a pretty campground, with many

RATINGS

Beauty: ✪ ✪ ✪ ✪
Privacy: ✪ ✪
Spaciousness: ✪ ✪
Quiet: ✪ ✪ ✪
Security: ✪ ✪ ✪ ✪ ✪
Cleanliness: ✪ ✪ ✪ ✪ ✪

of the sites following the natural contours of the land. It's also a heavily wooded camp-ground, and maintenance is impeccable. The Ash Loop (A) is nearest the entrance and visitor center and contains 32 sites (Site 2 reserved for camp host). A path heading to the lake sits between sites 11 and 13. Ash has six wheelchair-accessible sites (3 to 5 and 19 to 21). Next up is the Birch Loop (B) with 31 sites (sites 23 and 30 are reserved for camp hosts). There isn't much to distinguish the two loops except for the fact that Birch is home to an amphitheater. Again, this shouldn't be any concern at night, but daytime activities can make the sites nearest the amphitheater (specifically 24 and 25) feel like epicenters of commotion.

Skip the Cedar Loop (C) as its 41 sites are for RVs, with full electrical hookups. The final loop is Dogwood (D). Even though Dogwood is the most crowded, with 60 sites (sites 22 and 32 reserved for camp hosts), it's the farthest from the beach, lake, and camp-ground entrance. It's also a decent distance from the RV loop at Cedar. But it's also near-est hunting areas, so if you're camping during hunting season, you may hear some gunshots, though they will seem pretty far off. Sites 40 to 48, on the southern outside edge, offer the easiest access to the trails that access the AT; the same sites along the

KEY INFORMATION

ADDRESS:	Greenbrier State Park
	21843 National Pike
	Boonsboro, MD 21713-9535
	(301) 791-4767
OPERATED BY:	Maryland Department of Natural Resources
OPEN:	Late April–end of October
SITES:	165
EACH SITE HAS:	Picnic table, grill, lantern hook, tent pad
ASSIGNMENT:	Reservations required
REGISTRATION:	(888) 432-CAMP (2267) or at http://reservations.dnr.state.md.us
FACILITIES:	Picnic tables, grills, playgrounds, swimming beach, boat launch, boat rental, camp store, bathhouses, dump station
PARKING:	Vehicles must remain on gravel driveway
FEE:	$25/night, $30/night electric; half-price Sunday–Thursday for senior citizens; day-use service charge: Memorial Day–Labor Day, weekends and holidays $4/person, weekdays $3/person; May and September, weekends $3/person. Out-of-state residents add $1 to all day-use service charges.
RESTRICTIONS:	*Pets:* Not allowed
	Quiet Hours: 11 p.m.–7 a.m.
	Visitors: Max. 6 people
	Fires: In fire rings
	Alcohol: Not permitted at beach
	Stay Limit: 2 weeks
	Other: Check-out 3 p.m. There's one water pump in Ash, between sites 2 and 4; campers in other side of Ash might want to use Birch water pump, between sites 5 and 9

MAP

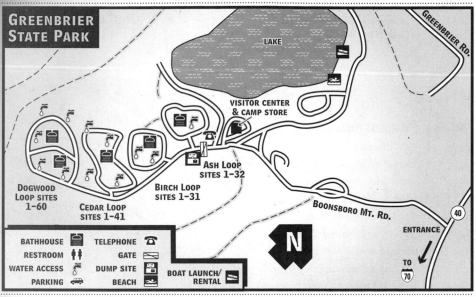

GREENBRIER STATE PARK

LAKE

VISITOR CENTER & CAMP STORE

ASH LOOP SITES 1-32

BIRCH LOOP SITES 1-31

DOGWOOD LOOP SITES 1-60

CEDAR LOOP SITES 1-41

BOONSBORO MT. RD.

GREENBRIER RD.

40

ENTRANCE

TO 70

BATHHOUSE		TELEPHONE	
RESTROOM		GATE	
WATER ACCESS		DUMP SITE	
PARKING		BEACH	

BOAT LAUNCH/ RENTAL

N

GETTING THERE

From the east: I-70 West to Exit 42, MD Route 17. Bear right onto Route 17 North. Turn left onto Route 40 West. Follow for 3 miles and the park is on the left. From the west: I-70 East to Exit 35, MD Route 66. Bear right onto 66. Turn left onto Route 40 East. Follow for 2 miles and the park is on the right.

western edge (24 to 38) offer easiest access to the hiking trails in the hunting area.

Greenbrier's campground is consistently well maintained and pretty. The only sites you may consider avoiding are those closest to the entrance road, as they sit pretty near the road: Ash: 1, 3, 5, 6, 8, 10, 26, 28, 30, 32; Birch: 1, 31; and Cedar: 1, 32, 33, 34, 36, 38, 40 (but you probably won't be in Cedar anyway). Dogwood is OK because the camp road ends there (or, more accurately, becomes the Dogwood Loop Road).

GPS COORDINATES

UTM Zone (NAD27) 18S
Easting 275507
Northing 4379721

19
MAPLE TREE CAMP

THE **APPALACHIAN MOUNTAIN** area surrounding the 20-acre Maple Tree Camp has a bit of unpleasant history, both real and fictional. Here, on South Mountain, more than 6,000 soldiers were killed in the Civil War, effectively ending Robert E. Lee's 1862 Maryland incursion. Some 140 years later, a fictional witch lurked in these parts, which served as the home of *The Blair Witch Project*. The popular film brought a steady stream of visitors to nearby Burkittsville (a real town without a witch), convinced of the story's veracity. The thick woods surrounding the town aren't illusory either, and they provide a great setting for one of Maryland's most unusual camping opportunities.

What attracts most to Maple Tree is the opportunity to sleep in a treehouse. Twelve such treehouses stud the property, nicely spaced from one another. Each treehouse is enclosed, sits seven feet off the ground, and has a small deck. The largest among them can accommodate up to ten people. In addition to the treehouses, there are tepees, a log cabin, wooded tent sites, and field sites.

Maple Tree's location makes it a strategic base from which to explore the immediate area, which offers no dearth of recreational activities. If you want history, Antietam National Battlefield—site of the single bloodiest battle in American history—and Harpers Ferry, West Virginia, are very close by (but do require a short drive to get there). If you want recreational activities, swimming and tubing on the Potomac are easy to do. Horseback riding can also be arranged at the camp office. If the weather is crummy, more options abound: go indoors to the fantastic Brunswick Railroad Museum in nearby Brunswick, or head underground where the weather doesn't change, at Crystal Grottoes Cavern just down the road from Antietam.

> *What attracts most to Maple Tree is the opportunity to sleep in a treehouse.*

RATINGS

Beauty: ☆ ☆ ☆ ☆
Privacy: ☆ ☆ ☆ ☆
Spaciousness: ☆ ☆ ☆ ☆ ☆
Quiet: ☆ ☆ ☆ ☆
Security: ☆ ☆ ☆ ☆ ☆
Cleanliness: ☆ ☆ ☆ ☆

ADDRESS: Maple Tree Camp
20716 Townsend
Road
Gapland, MD 21779
(301) 432-5585

OPERATED BY: Privately owned

OPEN: All year

SITES: 36 total (8 treehouses,
1 log cabin, 4 cot-
tages, 23 tent sites)

EACH SITE: Wooded tent sites:
fire circle, grill,
picnic table. Field
sites: picnic table,
fire circle

ASSIGNMENT: Reservations are
recommended and
are honored for up
to 4 days; 1-night
deposit required

REGISTRATION: Call (301) 432-5585 or
go to www.the
treehousecamp.com

FACILITIES: Bathhouses, camp
store, water, horse-
shoes, basketball
hoop, pavilion

PARKING: At designated sites

FEE: Wooded tent sites,
$10/person; field
tent sites, $8/person;
treehouses, $36/night
for up to 4 people,
$10 extra person

RESTRICTIONS: *Pets:* On leash
Quiet Hours: 11 p.m.–
7 a.m.
Visitors: Fee above
applies to all
overnight visitors
Fires: In fire rings
Alcohol: Permitted
Stay Limit: 2-night
minimum weekends,
except field sites;
3-night minimum
Memorial and Labor
Day weekends
Other: All sites 50%
off on Wednesday

Of course, the area offers great hiking opportunities. Greenbrier, Washington Monument, and Gathland State Parks are nearby, as is Devil's Backbone County Park, home to hiking and fishing in Antietam Creek under the shadows of a beautiful stone bridge that survived the Civil War. Best of all, a portion of the Appalachian Trail runs along the edge of the campground property. It's easily accessed and allows for great hiking. In fact, Maple Tree has become an increasingly popular stop for AT thru-hikers (it has hot showers, after all). Gathland State Park is just up the road from the turnoff used to get into Maple Tree; if for no other reason, a visit to see the Civil War Correspondent's Memorial is well worth the short hike there.

Best of all, Maple Tree does not allow RVs or trailers. It's quiet, and isolated, and the "wooded" tent sites are just that. Each, like the treehouses, affords a good amount of privacy and space. Tent sites range in size considerably; when you make reservations, specify how many tents you have, because different sites can accommodate anywhere from one to four tents. My favorite sites are those up the hill from the camp office, sitting more or less by themselves in thick woods and a pristine setting. Lion, Leopard, Otter, Badger, and Wildebeest are the first sites (grouped along a common entrance road); of these, Wildebeest, the last one reached, is the best, as it's completely isolated and has nothing but thick woods as its backyard. But beyond these sites, and beyond even the "End" sign on the road, are two wonderful, isolated sites: Hedgehog and Ram. These are my favorites. If you don't get a wooded site, or if you prefer to look up at the stars, field sites are situated just in front of the camp office.

I must admit that I didn't expect too much from Maple Tree Camp, as it could easily have relied on its reputation as a unique place and left it at that. But the campground is lovingly maintained by friendly and helpful owners, and it is truly a wonderful place, allowing for an easy getaway in an unspoiled setting. It's one of my favorites.

MAP

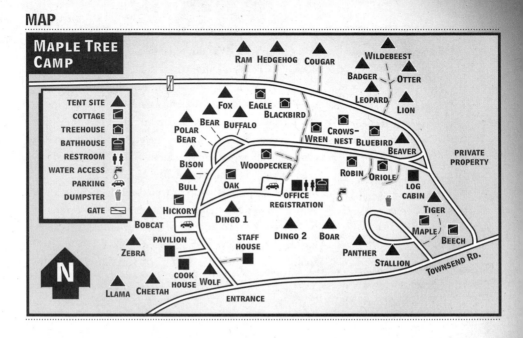

MAPLE TREE CAMP

Legend:
- TENT SITE
- COTTAGE
- TREEHOUSE
- BATHHOUSE
- RESTROOM
- WATER ACCESS
- PARKING
- DUMPSTER
- GATE

RAM · HEDGEHOG · COUGAR · WILDEBEEST
BADGER · OTTER · LEOPARD · LION
FOX · EAGLE · BLACKBIRD
BEAR · BUFFALO · CROWS-NEST · BLUEBIRD
POLAR BEAR · WREN · BEAVER
BISON · WOODPECKER · ROBIN · ORIOLE
BULL · OAK · OFFICE REGISTRATION · LOG CABIN
HICKORY · DINGO 1 · TIGER · MAPLE · BEECH
BOBCAT · STAFF HOUSE · DINGO 2 · BOAR · PANTHER
PAVILION · STALLION
ZEBRA · COOK HOUSE · WOLF
LLAMA · CHEETAH · ENTRANCE

PRIVATE PROPERTY

TOWNSEND RD.

N

GETTING THERE

Take I-70 to Frederick. Take
Exit 52, US 340 West and go
15 miles to MD Route 67
North toward Boonsboro.
Go 5 miles and turn right on
Gapland Road, then left on
Townsend Road.

GPS COORDINATES

UTM Zone (NAD27) 18S
Easting 272507
Northing 4365789

> *This is mountainous, unspoiled western Maryland—black bears, heavy snow, and all.*

NEW GERMANY SITS ON THE EASTERN side of the Continental Divide, but just barely. This makes it part of the Chesapeake watershed, a thought-provoking fact—if you're camping here, you'll feel a long way from Bay Country. This is mountainous, unspoiled western Maryland—black bears, heavy snow, and all. While it won't feel much like Chesapeake watershed, you probably won't be thinking of Germany either. The name of the area comes from the early settlers, who felt at home because of the landscape's similarity to the homes they left behind. Unfortunately, those same folks completely cleared the forest, as was custom in the 1800s. By the middle of the next century, however, the land was turned over to the state, and the CCC began improvements. Now the forests have been replanted, and some sections soar with century-old trees. In the park, the main attraction is 13-acre New Germany Lake, great for boating, fishing, and swimming. A result of damming Poplar Lick, New Germany Lake contains bass, catfish, tiger muskie, and trout. These same fish species, as well as walleye, can be reeled in from Poplar Lick.

Autumn comes a bit early in these higher elevations, so snagging a campsite at the end of the season is highly recommended. Aside from the lack of crowds, the fall foliage in the forest is simply spectacular. Gum, maple, and larch explode by October. Just remember if you're coming from eastern Maryland: the nights here get surprisingly cool.

The campground is wooded and private. There are 39 campsites on two loops, each sharing one bathhouse. The first loop is the Governor Thomas Loop, with sites 1 to 20 and 34 to 38. The Pine Loop is next, with sites 21 to 32 and 39. I really like Site 39 because it sits by itself at the end of what appears to be a small gravel driveway. There's one potential catch,

RATINGS

Beauty: ✿ ✿ ✿ ✿
Privacy: ✿ ✿ ✿
Quiet: ✿ ✿ ✿
Spaciousness: ✿ ✿ ✿
Security: ✿ ✿ ✿ ✿ ✿
Cleanliness: ✿ ✿ ✿ ✿

however—a short trail behind it leads to a parking lot. If people mistake this for a forest trail, you might get some company. It might be worth the chance, however, as it's easily the most private spot in the campground. I also prefer the Pine Loop in general; as its name indicates, it's studded with pines and the aroma is wonderful.

Sites 33 and 34 are very close together, and 36 sits right next to the bathhouse. Site 28 is nice, as it backs to thick woods. If stargazing is your thing, go for 29, which is very open. Mostly every site is acceptable and promises quiet, as none are electric. For campers needing electricity, there are ten camper cabins, all of them behind the nature center on a separate road from the camp loops. Cabin 3 is wheelchair accessible. If you get caught by bad weather but begrudge going into the camper cabin, there are three-sided alpine-style shelters just up the road from sites 30 and 32.

Generally speaking, you'll be able to get a spot in New Germany if you're just popping in. Aside from four nonreservable sites (29 to 32), the overflow area allows for nine more camping sites. Trying to accommodate campers seems more the rule than the exception at New Germany. That said, a reservation is never a bad idea.

KEY INFORMATION

ADDRESS: New Germany State Park 349 Headquarters Lane Grantsville, MD 21536 (301) 895-5453

OPERATED BY: Maryland Department of Natural Resources

OPEN: Last weekend in April–September 1; overflow area until mid-October

SITES: 39, plus 9 overflow near park entrance

EACH SITE HAS: Picnic table, lantern post, grill, camp pad

ASSIGNMENT: First come, first served early September–end of the season; reservations recommended otherwise

REGISTRATION: (888) 432-CAMP (2267) or at http://reservations.dnr.state.md.us

FACILITIES: Bathhouses (no showers early September–end of season), boat rental, nature center, playground

PARKING: 2 vehicles per site

FEE: $20/night; Memorial Day–Labor Day weekends and holidays, $2/person day-use fee

RESTRICTIONS: *Pets:* Prohibited
Quiet Hours: 11 p.m.–7 a.m.
Visitors: Max. 6 people per site
Fires: In fire rings
Alcohol: At site only
Stay Limit: 2 weeks

MAP

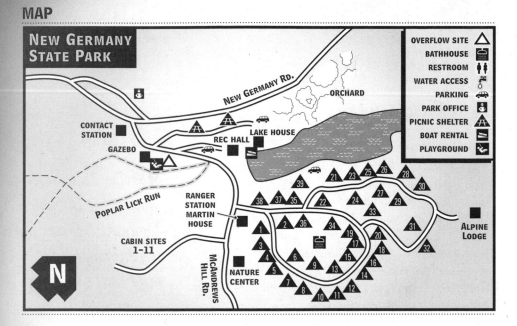

GETTING THERE

Take Exit 22 off I-68 and follow Chestnut Ridge Road south to New Germany Road.

GPS COORDINATES

UTM Zone (NAD27) 17S
Easting 661351
Northing 4388758

21
POTOMAC
STATE FOREST:
LOSTLAND RUN AREA AND
BACKCOUNTRY CAMPING

THE **POTOMAC STATE FOREST** is a special place, as it retains the vestiges of the wildness that used to make Western Maryland the first frontier for expansion-minded colonials. While the Allegheny Range of the Appalachian Mountains is puny by western standards, the mountains proved a formidable obstacle to many heading west.

A friend of mine from Colorado scoffs at Maryland's "mountains," but I love my Appalachians. They are beautiful, rolling mountains, older by many centuries than the Rockies. Maryland's tallest mountain, Backbone Mountain, forms the northwest ridge of the land that comprises Potomac State Forest. The summit of Backbone (3,360 feet) is farther to the southeast, near the West Virginia border. But the ridge runs north, spilling its rainwater and snowmelt along several "runs" as they make their way to the Potomac River, some 1,000 feet below.

One of these waterways is the Lostland Run, which, along with the North Hill area, gives its name to Potomac State Forest's northern sections. In the Lostland Run Area, there's some great camping for those who want to get away from it all.

Following the directions, when you reach the Potomac Resource Center (Ranger Station), you will pass the trailhead for the Lostland Run Trail. This trail winds all the way to the incredible Potomac Overlook. It also winds close to each of the camping areas, paralleling the unpaved Lostland Run Road and traversing both the South Prong (of the Lostland Run) and North Prong suspension bridges. The trail is easily accessible from any of the five camping sites (plus one group site) in this area.

To get to the campsites, pass the headquarters of the Potomac Resource Center; take note of the picnic areas, bathrooms, and water nearby. Farther along

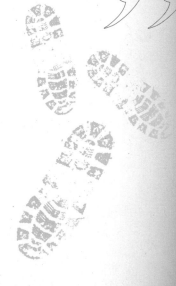

> *Maryland's tallest mountain, Backbone Mountain, forms the northwest ridge of the land that comprises Potomac State Forest.*

RATINGS

Beauty: ✰ ✰ ✰ ✰ ✰
Privacy: ✰ ✰ ✰ ✰ ✰
Spaciousness: ✰ ✰ ✰ ✰ ✰
Quiet: ✰ ✰ ✰ ✰ ✰
Security: ✰ ✰ ✰
Cleanliness: ✰ ✰ ✰ ✰ ✰

ADDRESS: Potomac-Garrett
State Forest
222 Herrington Lane
Oakland, MD 21550
(301) 334-2038

OPERATED BY: Maryland Department of Natural
Resources

OPEN: All year, but roads
are not maintained
in winter

SITES: 6+ (6 in Lostland Run
Area, unlimited in
forest backcountry)

EACH SITE HAS: Lantern hook, grill,
picnic table (Lost-
land Run Area)

ASSIGNMENT: First come, first
served; group sites
must be reserved

REGISTRATION: Self-registration stations at the entrance
to each area; to
reserve a group site,
call (301) 334-2038.

FACILITIES: Group sites have
sanitation facilities
but no potable water

PARKING: Vehicles must be
parked on gravel
portion of site, off
road in forest

FEE: $10/night, $15 lean-
to shelter, $20 group

RESTRICTIONS: *Pets:* Permitted
Quiet Hours: 11 p.m.–
7 a.m.
Visitors: Max. 8 peo-
ple/2 units (20 peo-
ple for group sites)
Fires: In fire rings
Alcohol: Permitted
Stay Limit: 2 weeks
Other: Check-out is 3
p.m. for roadside
sites. This is bear
country; take precau-
tions. Camping is
prohibited within
200 feet of any trail
or stream.

Potomac Camp Road, you'll see the unpaved Lostland Run Road to the right. The self-registration station is just up ahead. The first site along the road is 30. Like all the established sites in the state forest, it's spacious, private, and set in a beautiful natural setting—you can't go wrong with any of the sites along the road. Which you choose should depend mostly on vacancy and how much bumpy driving you're willing to endure to make your way along Lostland Run Road.

As part of a group site, there is another picnic area (marked T-35) and toilet just beyond Site 30; Site 31 is just ahead as well. Then it's a good distance to the next site, more than 0.8 miles. Again, it's a jarring ride down the unpaved road, and even though getting closer to the river might be desirable, taking the trail there on foot is the much more pleasurable way to arrive. However, it might be worth the car trip down this road because just after Site 32 is a lean-to shelter site; like the same in the other sections of the Potomac State Forest (see page 75), these sites are well worth the extra five dollars. If you're suddenly hit with a deluge during the night, it's nice to have the luxury of settling into the shelter.

If you're still making your way down Lostland Run Road and you've passed the shelter, you only have one more choice for a campsite, Site 34. I wouldn't expect all the sites to be taken, as this area is pretty remote. However, if you find this is the case—or you want an even more backcountry experience—you are allowed to camp in any primitive setting in the state forest, so long as you don't pitch your tent within 200 feet of a trail or stream. Backcountry permits can be obtained through the self-registration stations at Lostland Run or Laurel Run/Wallman (see page 75).

If you do desire backcountry camping, you can either venture off the main arteries described above, or into the North Hill area, a wild and rugged section of the state forest north of Lostland Run. To reach it, stay on Potomac Camp Road, passing the turnoff for the Lostland Run area, and follow Potomac Camp to a right on North Hill Road. Be on the lookout about 0.2 miles later for the North Hill Trail, a small tertiary road. Once here, you'll find places to leave the car

POTOMAC STATE FOREST:
LOSTLAND RUN AREA
AND BACKCOUNTRY CAMPING

POTOMAC CAMP RD.
NORTH PRONG
POTOMAC CAMP RD.
CCC FISH REARING PONDS TRAIL
N
3D ARCHERY RANGE
EAGLE SCOUT TRAIL
POTOMAC CAMP RD.
HUBBARD RD.
COMBINATION RD.
LOSTLAND RUN
LOSTLAND RUN TRAIL
LOSTLAND RUN RD.
POTOMAC OVERLOOK
CASCADE FALLS
NORTH BRANCH POTOMAC RIVER

CAMPSITE ▲	SHELTER	
RESTROOM	OVERLOOK △	
WATER ACCESS	PARK OFFICE	
PARKING	FALLS	
PICNIC AREA	FISHING	

(take care not to block the passage) and set off into deep, untamed, unmarked forest.

There are two more forest areas ripe for backcountry camping. Following the directions above for North Hill, you can bypass North Hill Road and instead head left onto Upperman Road. When Upperman intersects with Eagle Rock Road, take a left; this quadrant of forest, to the south and east, is all prime camping area. Last, the Wallman Area (see page 76) runs pretty far south of the main campsites. Loop Road, Bradshaw Hollow Road, and Trestle Road (nearest the Potomac) can all be accessed by heading south from Wallman Road, and you can camp in the forest anywhere off these roads.

GETTING THERE

From Oakland, take MD Route 135 East to MD Route 560 and turn right. Go 3 miles to a left on Bethlehem Road. (Stay on Bethlehem at the intersection to Eagle Rock Road). Go left on Combination Road and left on Potomac Camp Road. Pass the Potomac Resource Center, and the self-registration station is on Lostland Run Road.

GPS COORDINATES

UTM Zone (NAD27) 17S
Easting 648306
Northing 4360544

22
POTOMAC STATE FOREST:
LAUREL RUN AND WALLMAN AREAS

The cliffs that overlook the Potomac are impressive and offer endless opportunities for sightseeing.

THE POTOMAC STATE FOREST encompasses more than 11,000 acres of pristine wilderness bordering the North Branch of the Potomac River. The forest also includes portions of Backbone Mountain, Maryland's highest point. While the summit of Backbone sits outside of the state forest, sections within the forest exceed 3,000 feet. Both the Wallman and Laurel Run areas maintain elevation levels of 2,000 to 2,700 feet.

Like much of Maryland's western forests, the entire area was once denuded but has been allowed to grow back naturally and now serves as a protected area for an abundance of wildlife, including a thriving population of black bears. There are well-marked trails all throughout this rugged mountain wilderness; the state forest provides for some ideal backcountry camping. The cliffs that overlook the Potomac are impressive and offer endless opportunities for sightseeing.

Follow the directions, and when Audley Riley Road loses its pavement you'll see the self-registration station. The road splits here; left is Laurel Run Road, right is Wallman Road, both unpaved.

Laurel Run Road heads east and ends at a fishing spot on the North Branch of the Potomac River. Because of the condition of the road, it makes for a long drive. Be prepared for the jarring the unpaved roads will inflict on your car. You might be tempted to stop at the first campsite you come to so as to avoid more jarring. This wouldn't be such a terrible thing. The first site, T-20, is a good indicator of the campsites all along Laurel Run Road—spacious, roomy, and in a beautiful setting. Your only reason for venturing beyond this site is if it's already taken, or if you wish to be nearer the river. If you want to push on, the next site, 21, is the only one of the ten sites along Laurel Run Road that has a lean-to shelter. Built in 2000 and

RATINGS

Beauty: ✰ ✰ ✰ ✰ ✰
Privacy: ✰ ✰ ✰ ✰ ✰
Spaciousness: ✰ ✰ ✰ ✰ ✰
Quiet: ✰ ✰ ✰ ✰ ✰
Security: ✰ ✰ ✰
Cleanliness: ✰ ✰ ✰ ✰ ✰

called the Laurel Run Lodge (a bit of a misnomer), it's solidly constructed and still new. If there's a chance of horrendous weather, why not give yourself the security of having the shelter to duck into if need be? Even if you never use the shelter, the site itself is extraordinary. Laurel Run (a beautiful rocky river) flows just behind the site, along with a narrow hiking trail.

After that, the sites are more or less the same—roomy, private, and in a spectacular natural setting; you really can't go wrong with any one of them. Be aware that while the first three campsites come relatively quickly one after the other (assuming you're traveling by car), the next one (site 22) is half a mile away. It is followed very quickly by sites 23, 24, and 25, which also sit near one another, about a tenth of a mile farther east on Laurel Run Road. There are two more sites along the road, the last one (site 27) about half a mile from the river.

Back at the self-registration station, if you had headed right along Wallman Road, the first thing you come to is a large group camping site (40). It is followed by two picnic areas, another group site, and a bathroom off Loop Road; Loop Road eventually heads deep into the wilds of the forested Wallman Area. You'll notice that the group sites are not that much bigger than the single sites. Beyond the group sites, there are four more campsites, all in relatively quick succession. The third one is a shelter site like the one in the Laurel Run section described above; if it's available I would grab it.

Of the two areas, I prefer Laurel Run over Wallman, as it feels a bit more wooded to me. If you want river access, Laurel Run is the better option as well. Where Wallman Road makes a sharp right after the final campsite, there's a parking area straight ahead and a Disabled Hunter Access Road that leads to Trestle Road (all unpaved). You'd have to take a left on Trestle and make your way to Laurel Run Road to get down to the river.

My preference for Laurel Run is a subjective one—the truth is that camping in the Potomac State Forest is fantastic wherever you wind up. If you're looking for an accessible backcountry camping experience, you're sure to enjoy it.

KEY INFORMATION

ADDRESS: Potomac-Garrett State Forest 222 Herrington Lane Oakland, MD 21550 (301) 334-2038

OPERATED BY: Maryland Department of Natural Resources

OPEN: All year, but roads are not maintained in winter

SITES: 16 (10 at Laurel Run, 6 at Wallman)

EACH SITE HAS: Lantern hook, grill, picnic table

ASSIGNMENT: First come, first served; group sites must be reserved

REGISTRATION: Self-registration stations at the entrance to each area; to reserve a group site, call (301) 334-2038.

FACILITIES: Group sites have sanitation facilities but no potable water.

PARKING: Vehicles must be parked on gravel portion of site.

FEE: $10/night, $15 lean-to shelter, $20 group

RESTRICTIONS: *Pets:* Permitted *Quiet Hours:* 11 p.m.–7 a.m. *Visitors:* Max. 8 people/2 units (20 people for group sites) *Fires:* In fire rings *Alcohol:* Permitted *Stay Limit:* 2 weeks *Other:* Check-out is 3 p.m. This is bear country; take proper precautions.

MAP

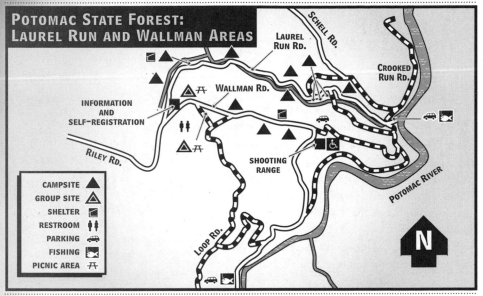

GETTING THERE

From Oakland, take MD Route 135 East to MD Route 560 and turn right. Go 3.5 miles to a left on White Church-Steyer Road. Go left on Audley Riley Road to the self-registration station.

GPS COORDINATES

UTM Zone (NAD27) 17S
Easting 646952
Northing 4355979

ROCKY GAP STATE PARK'S official name is Rocky Gap State Park and Lodge Resort, hinting at the monstrosity that sits there (of course, whether big is bad depends upon your view). The resort, complete with a hotel, Jack Nicklaus golf course, and restaurants, was the brainchild of an Allegany County congressman. Its intent was to draw tourists and create jobs, but this hasn't quite worked out. Year after year, the resort struggles to make money.

A hemlock stand within the gorge is a sight to behold.

The park itself contains more than 3,000 acres, including 243-acre Lake Habeeb. Many first-time campers at Rocky Gap seeking to get away from it all are horrified when they enter the park and see the sprawling complex before them. Take heart: planners had the good sense to at least build the resort and golf course on the other side of Lake Habeeb from the campgrounds. So, although you have to drive through the resort area to get to your campsite, once there you will enjoy relative solitude (as much as a campground with 278 sites can offer).

Even better, hiking away from the lake will leave all the bustle behind and you'll likely cross very few people as you make your way around Evitts Mountain, named for the settler who built his cabin here in the 1730s. When my buddy Jack and I camped and hiked here, we met my father and walked along the Evitts Mountain Homesite Trail, enjoying thick forest and canyon overlooks along the way. True, it was raining, but it was high season and we walked for five hours without seeing one other person. Unfortunately, we didn't see any black bears or bobcats either, but they're out there, along with the more common white-tailed deer and red fox. Two 500-acre tracts have been designated as state wildlands and are truly beautiful. A hemlock stand within the gorge is also a site to behold.

Rocky Gap has nine camp loops, each corresponding to its first letter—A for Ash, B for Birch, C for

RATINGS

Beauty: ✩ ✩ ✩ ✩
Privacy: ✩ ✩ ✩
Spaciousness: ✩ ✩ ✩
Quiet: ✩ ✩
Security: ✩ ✩ ✩ ✩
Cleanliness: ✩ ✩ ✩ ✩ ✩

Chestnut, etc. The others: Dogwood, Elm, Fir, Gum, Hickory, and Ironwood. Ash, with its 30 sites, is electric and allows pets. Birch, Chestnut, and Dogwood all intersect and are all very close to one another. While individual sites are often separated by 50 or more feet of nice tree buffers, don't expect to feel alone in any of these loops unless you're here mid-week or in the off-season. If you do stay in one of these three loops (bathhouses are within Dogwood and Chestnut), I'd recommend the western edge of Dogwood (pet loop also), specifically sites 91 and 92 or those close by. These sites are bounded by woods (the other side of the loop is bounded by Chestnut) and sit astride the wonderful Evitts Mountain Homesite Trail. It means that if you didn't feel alone, you can take a few steps and achieve solitude.

Elm Loop (sites 11 to 143) offers easy access to the camp store and sits near the lake, so if water sports are more your thing, this might be a good option. It's also closest to the Lakeside Loop Trail, a challenging and rewarding path around the shoreline. Sites 120 to 125 are closest to the lake. Gum (sites 175 to 204) and Hickory (sites 205 to 237) are next; you can find very accommodating tent sites here, but they are blocked from the water by Fir and Ironwood. The southern sites in Hickory (232 to 237) are near the group camping area. Consequently, these can be noisier than others. Sites 220 to 228 on the northwest corner of Hickory also provide easy access to the southern portion of the Evitts Mountain Homesite Trail.

KEY INFORMATION

ADDRESS:	Rocky Gap State Park
	12500 Pleasant Valley Road
	Flintstone, MD 21530
	(301) 722-1480
OPERATED BY:	Maryland Department of Natural Resources
OPEN:	First weekend in April–Labor Day; select loops open until mid-December
SITES:	278
EACH SITE HAS:	Picnic table, fire ring
ASSIGNMENT:	First come, first served in select loops from Labor Day–mid-December; reservations recommended otherwise
REGISTRATION:	(888) 432-CAMP (2267) or online at www.reservations.dnr.state.md.us
FACILITIES:	Dump station, bathhouses, boat ramp and rentals, laundry, camp store, nature center, game room, swimming beach, pay phones
PARKING:	On gravel driveway
FEE:	$25/night, $30/night electric, $225/night family group site (max. 40 people); day-use service charge: Memorial Day–Labor Day weekdays, $2/vehicle; Memorial Day–Labor Day weekends and holidays, $5/vehicle; boat launch, $5/vehicle; out-of-state residents, add $1 to all service charges
RESTRICTIONS:	*Pets:* Allowed in Ash and Dogwood loops
	Quiet Hours: 11 p.m.–7 a.m.
	Visitors: Check-in at registration desk
	Fires: In fire rings
	Alcohol: Permitted
	Stay Limit: Max. 10 consecutive days
	Other: Check-out 3 p.m.

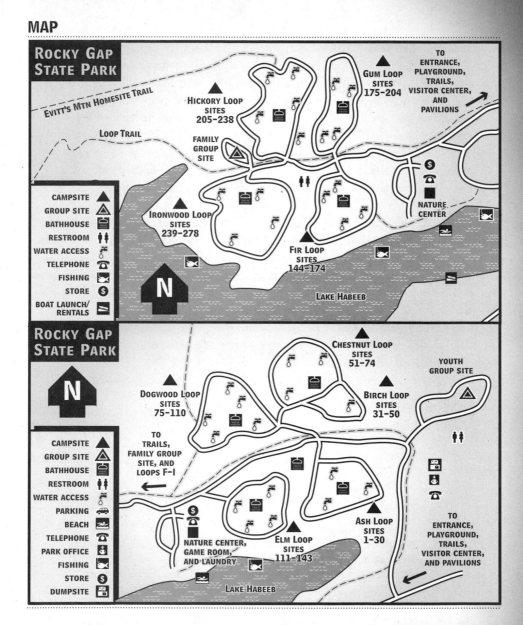

ROCKY GAP STATE PARK

EVITT'S MTN HOMESITE TRAIL

LOOP TRAIL

HICKORY LOOP
SITES
205–238

GUM LOOP
SITES
175–204

TO
ENTRANCE,
PLAYGROUND,
TRAILS,
VISITOR CENTER,
AND
PAVILIONS

FAMILY
GROUP
SITE

NATURE
CENTER

IRONWOOD LOOP
SITES
239–278

FIR LOOP
SITES
144–174

LAKE HABEEB

CAMPSITE
GROUP SITE
BATHHOUSE
RESTROOM
WATER ACCESS
TELEPHONE
FISHING
STORE
BOAT LAUNCH/
RENTALS

N

ROCKY GAP STATE PARK

N

CHESTNUT LOOP
SITES
51–74

YOUTH
GROUP SITE

DOGWOOD LOOP
SITES
75–110

BIRCH LOOP
SITES
31–50

TO
TRAILS,
FAMILY GROUP
SITE, AND
LOOPS F–I

CAMPSITE
GROUP SITE
BATHHOUSE
RESTROOM
WATER ACCESS
PARKING
BEACH
TELEPHONE
PARK OFFICE
FISHING
STORE
DUMPSITE

NATURE CENTER,
GAME ROOM,
AND LAUNDRY

ELM LOOP
SITES
111–143

ASH LOOP
SITES
1–30

TO
ENTRANCE,
PLAYGROUND,
TRAILS,
VISITOR CENTER,
AND PAVILIONS

LAKE HABEEB

Lastly, Fir (sites 144 to 174) and Ironwood (239 to 278) are often the most popular because of their proximity to Lake Habeeb. Sites 156 to 166 in Fir and 255 to 265 in Ironwood are closest to the lake, with 256 to 260 nearest the dock. Ironwood also offers easy access to the Lakeside Loop Trail, which is the most popular in the park. Again, my recommendation is to head farther away from the lake and toward the less used, more pleasant trails. You can always check out the lake after you're down from the mountain.

GETTING THERE

Take I-68 to Exit 50 (Rocky Gap State Park).

GPS COORDINATES

UTM Zone (NAD27) 17S
Easting 701709
Northing 4398306

> *What makes the campsites in the state forest unique is that most guarantee almost total privacy.*

THINGS CAN GET A BIT CONFUSING in these parts, with so many competing parks (including Big Run, page 10 and New Germany, page 69) and recreation areas, all contained within the 54,000-acre Savage River Forest. What makes the campsites in the state forest unique is that most guarantee almost total privacy. The Savage River sites sit spread like tentacles near and around Big Run and New Germany state parks and the Savage River Reservoir. Savage River Forest is Maryland's largest protected site, and it includes some 12,000 acres of wildlands, which earn special protections. There are some 100 miles of trails throughout the forest, allowing you to pick a length and configuration and go.

Fishing and boating are also popular in the forest. Interestingly, its two main rivers, Savage and Casselman, end up in very different places: Savage heads to the Potomac and eventually ends up in the Atlantic, while Casselman sits on the western side of the continental divide, heads to the Youghiogheny, and eventually empties its waters in the Mississippi. Many regard these rivers and native trout streams as the best trout fisheries in the state.

The reservoir itself is a major draw and sees many boaters and anglers. But the forest's location in a relatively remote portion of the state assures that it never feels overrun. I've split the forest camping into two entries in this book because of the differing nature of each. This entry covers the area northeast of the reservoir, between the reservoir and New Germany State Park. In this mountainous, wooded location you won't be very near the reservoir itself but will have easy access to the pristine forest. The campsites located here provide a year-round and inexpensive alternative to New Germany. Plus, compared to New Germany, the Savage River sites give a more backcountry, remote feel to your

RATINGS

Beauty: ✩ ✩ ✩ ✩
Privacy: ✩ ✩ ✩ ✩ ✩
Spaciousness: ✩ ✩ ✩ ✩
Quiet: ✩ ✩ ✩ ✩
Security: ✩ ✩ ✩
Cleanliness: ✩ ✩ ✩ ✩

camping experience. While amenities like those at New Germany are nice, for me the seclusion of the Savage River State Forest campsites beats a maintained campground any day.

Campsites in this section are spread along Westernport Road in the Elk Lick Area and along the Poplar Lick ORV Trail heading south toward Savage River Road and the reservoir. First, Poplar Lick: If you were heading south along New Germany Road from New Germany State Park and the state forest headquarters, you'd soon see a little dirt road just after the New Germany store. A sign there indicates Poplar Lick ORV Trail. The first site you'll come to, on the left, is Site 135. Another 15 sites (134 to 120) follow the trail until it reaches Savage River Road. These are nice sites, much like the state forest campsites at Garrett and Potomac—generally a cleared space in the forest just off the road or trail and studded with trees. They are large, very private, and well wooded. In the case of the Poplar Lick sites, the little waterway sits just behind the sites with the exception of 134, 122, and 123, which are on the right side of the trail/road heading south. There is one reason for hesitation when it comes to these sites, however—this is an ORV trail, and off-road vehicles can mean noise. Although ORVs (trucks and vehicles with four- or all-wheel drive) are less noisy and smelly than ATVs (all-terrain vehicles) any passing vehicle's capacity for spoiling

KEY INFORMATION

ADDRESS: Savage River State Forest
127 Headquarters Lane
Grantsville, MD 21536
(301) 895-5759

OPERATED BY: Maryland Department of Natural Resources

OPEN: All year

SITES: 26, plus back-country camping

EACH SITE HAS: Picnic table, fire ring, tent pad

ASSIGNMENT: First come, first served

REGISTRATION: Self-register within first hour of arrival by taking green envelope, putting in money, and filling out form; place form in one of the green self-registration standpipes found on Savage River Road southeast of the reservoir, Elk Lick Run on Westernport Road, the southern edge of the Poplar Lick ORV Trail, at BJ's store on Savage River Road, on Big Run Road at the whitewater campgrounds below Savage River Reservoir, at the Savage River shooting range off New Germany Road, and the Savage River State Headquarters.

FACILITIES: Boat launches, supplies at BJ's store

PARKING: Max. 2 vehicles per site; must be parked in entrance drive or camping pad

FEE: $10/night numbered sites, $5/night backcountry

RESTRICTIONS: *Pets:* Permitted on a leash
Quiet Hours: 11 p.m.–7 a.m.
Visitors: Max. 6 people and 2 tents per site
Fires: Allowed in fire rings but not within the 12,000 acres of the Wildlands areas if backcountry camping; consult a park map available at headquarters
Alcohol: Permitted
Stay Limit: Each numbered site must be reserved daily
Other: This is bear country; for tips on how to camp among bears, visit www.dnr.state.md.us/wildlife/bbmd.html.

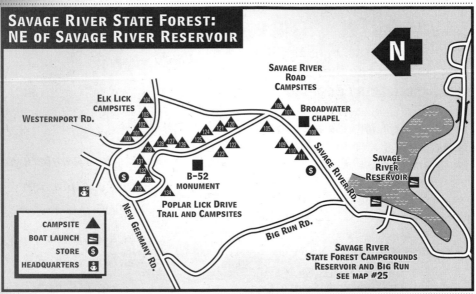

SAVAGE RIVER STATE FOREST:
NE OF SAVAGE RIVER RESERVOIR

GETTING THERE

To Savage River State Forest
Headquarters: Take I-68 to
Exit 22, US 219 toward
Meyersdale. Turn left onto
Chestnut Ridge Road/US
219. Continue on Chestnut
Ridge. Turn left onto New
Germany Road. Turn right
onto Headquarters Lane.

GPS COORDINATES

UTM Zone (NAD27) 17S
Easting 658936
Northing 4386305

your solitude and peacefulness depends entirely upon
the driver's speed and general courtesy.

Closer to New Germany State Park are the five
sites along Westernport Road, which you can reach by
following the directions to New Germany State Park
and then either going through the park on McAn-
drews Hill Road or just north of the park on Twin
Churches Road and then heading right (south) on
Westernport. The campsites (100 to 104) sit along
Westernport just before you reach Savage River Road.
These sites are much easier to get to than those along
the Poplar Lick Trail, so if you have a smallish vehicle,
these might be your better bets. Further, because of
their proximity to Savage River Road (what consti-
tutes a "major" road in these parts), you can easily
access the reservoir. Even better in this regard would
be the last sites in this section (105 to 111). You'll find
them along Savage River Road just after passing the
southern terminus of the Poplar Lick Trail. Their
advantage is easy access to the reservoir and BJ's
store, just south on Savage River Road. Of these sites,
those on the left side of the road (106 to 108) are the
nicest, as they sit near Savage River.

25
SAVAGE RIVER STATE FOREST: RESERVOIR AND BIG RUN NORTH (PLUS HUNTING SITES AND BACKCOUNTRY CAMPING)

NOTE: **THE RATINGS FOR PRIVACY,** spaciousness, and quiet are knocked down one star because of the sites along Savage River Road to the southeast of the reservoir, thus the parentheses. If you camp at any of the sites along Big Run Road, the privacy, spaciousness, and quiet ratings all go up a star.

As explained in the previous entry, I've split the Savage River State Forest camping into two for this book: this entry assumes that you've entered the state forest campsites from the southeast of the reservoir, along Savage River Road. Such a route provides camping near the river and reservoir and follows a route south of the reservoir, through Big Run State Park (see page 10), and then north along Big Run Road.

The campsite numbering system is a bit confusing. Existing maps show the campsites along Savage River Road as 112 to 119, but when I camped in the forest and checked out these sites, they were numbered 170 to 179, east to west. A very helpful ranger explained to me that the rangers' office recently added two sites here and then renumbered them all. These sites are popular, as they sit very near the reservoir and offer easy access to the boat launch on its southern end. Also, they're easy to get to, as Savage River Road is paved and the sites sit right off the road. However, they don't offer much privacy because they sit near one another and aren't very heavily wooded.

Continuing around the reservoir along Savage River Road (an absolutely beautiful ride, which will undoubtedly compel you to stop the car and head down to the water), you'll reach Big Run State Park (see page 10). Here is another boat launch, and then come the rest of the state forest sites along Big Run Road as it heads north to New Germany Road. The sites here begin with 149 and go to 136 in descending order. In comparison to the 170s, these sites are much

> *Negro Mountain has an elevation over 3,000 feet and was named in the 18th century in honor of an African-American fighter in the French and Indian War.*

RATINGS

Beauty: ☆ ☆ ☆ ☆ ☆
Privacy: ☆ ☆ ☆ ☆ (☆)
Spaciousness: ☆ ☆ ☆ (☆)
Quiet: ☆ ☆ ☆ ☆ (☆)
Security: ☆ ☆ ☆ ☆
Cleanliness: ☆ ☆ ☆ ☆ ☆

bigger, more private (often enjoying a couple hundred feet or more between them), and sit within thick forest. Because Big Run Road is also a paved road, these sites are easy to access and offer a wonderful camping experience that feels much more remote than in nearby Big Run State Park.

In discussing the above numbering issue with the ranger, I asked about what seemed to be some missing campsites: 150 to 169. He tipped me off to two more camping areas within the forest, both of which are, in his words, "seldom used because they lack access to water." They are primitive and remote. Additionally, these sites don't show up on campground maps. They are used primarily by deer hunters but are accessible and fall under the same rules and procedures as the rest of the sites within the forest. These sites are found in two different locations. The first location (sites 150 to 159) can be accessed off I-68, Exit 19 (US 219 South). Go about 2 miles to a left on Rabbit Hollow Road, where the sites are located. This area is called the Margraff Trails area, used mostly by hunters from nearby Accident. The other location is at Keysers Ridge, on Negro Mountain (elevation more than 3,000 feet and named in the 18th century in honor of an African-American fighter in the French and Indian War). It can also be reached by taking

KEY INFORMATION

ADDRESS: **Savage River State Forest**
127 Headquarters Lane
Grantsville, MD 21536
(301) 895-5759

OPERATED BY: **Maryland Department of Natural Resources**

OPEN: **All year**

SITES: **24, plus 19 hunting sites and backcountry camping**

EACH SITE HAS: **Picnic table, fire ring, tent pad**

ASSIGNMENT: **First come, first served**

REGISTRATION: **Self-register within first hour of arrival by taking green envelope, putting in money, and filling out form; place form in one of the green self-registration standpipes found on Savage River Road southeast of the reservoir, Elk Lick Run on Westernport Road, the southern edge of the Poplar Lick ORV Trail, at BJ's store on Savage River Road, on Big Run Road at the whitewater campgrounds below Savage River Reservoir, at the Savage River shooting range off New Germany Road, or the Savage River State Headquarters.**

FACILITIES: **Boat launches, supplies at BJ's Store**

PARKING: **Max. 2 vehicles per site; vehicles must be parked in entrance drive or camping pad**

FEE: **$10/night numbered sites, $5/night backcountry**

RESTRICTIONS: *Pets:* **Permitted on a leash**
Quiet Hours: **11 p.m.–7 a.m.**
Visitors: **Max. 6 people and 2 tents per site**
Fires: **Allowed in fire rings but not within the 12,000 acres of the Wildlands areas if backcountry camping**
Alcohol: **Permitted**
Stay Limit: **Each numbered site must be reserved daily**
Other: **This is bear country; for tips on how to camp among bears, visit www.dnr.state.md.us/wildlife/bbmd.html.**

MAP

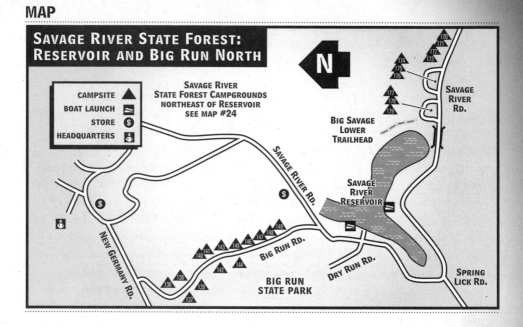

**SAVAGE RIVER STATE FOREST:
RESERVOIR AND BIG RUN NORTH**

N

CAMPSITE ▲
BOAT LAUNCH
STORE $
HEADQUARTERS

SAVAGE RIVER
STATE FOREST CAMPGROUNDS
NORTHEAST OF RESERVOIR
SEE MAP #24

SAVAGE
RIVER
RD.

BIG SAVAGE
LOWER
TRAILHEAD

SAVAGE RIVER RD.

SAVAGE
RIVER
RESERVOIR

NEW GERMANY RD.

BIG RUN RD.

DRY RUN RD.

SPRING
LICK RD.

BIG RUN
STATE PARK

Exit 14, but going north instead to US 40 West. Look for Keysers Ridge Road as a dirt track north (right) of US 40. Here, you'll find sites 160 to 169.

You can also camp anywhere in the state forest beyond the numbered sites. You must follow the same rules as those that apply to the numbered sites. To do so, register as you would for the numbered sites and include a trip itinerary and the names of the people in your camping party. Also, make sure to heed the restriction against fires within the 12,000 acres of the Wildlands areas. These areas are not contiguous and it's very important that you consult a map to make sure you know whether your camp sits within the parameters of the protected areas.

GETTING THERE

To Savage River Road southeast of the reservoir: I-68 to Exit 34, MD Route 36 (New Georges Creek Road) south to Luke. Go west on MD 135 and head right (northwest) onto Savage River Road. To Savage River State Forest Headquarters: see previous entry.

GPS COORDINATES

UTM Zone (NAD27) 17S
Easting 660924
Northing 4374247

26
SOUTH MOUNTAIN STATE PARK:
APPALACHIAN TRAIL SHELTERS

> *The great ideal of the AT is its accessibility to everyone willing to give it a go.*

THE APPALACHIAN TRAIL is blazed in white; blue blazes indicate trails to the Maryland shelters where you can pitch your tent. Prominent signage makes finding the shelters very easy.

I must confess that I was very hesitant about including AT entries in this book. On one hand, I have a strong feeling that the campsites described here and in the next entry should be the sole domain of Appalachian Trail thru-hikers. After all, if you're undertaking that difficult trek, it's not unreasonable to expect that the relatively few campsites in the area should be reserved for you as opposed to folks who've simply driven in somewhere close by and want to set up for the night. (South Mountain State Park doesn't advertise itself as a camping destination; the understanding is that the six primitive shelters and camping areas within the park are for AT thru-hikers.) But then I thought it over: the great ideal of the AT is its accessibility to everyone willing to give it a go. True, perhaps one who has hiked from Maine and eventually arrives in Maryland should have dibs on the campsites, but there's nothing wrong with locals who are hiking just the Maryland section, no small undertaking in itself, at over 40 miles. (My assumption is that Marylanders who are hiking the entire AT are aware of what campsites are where and wouldn't necessarily look to this book to provide the info.)

Ultimately, I decided to include the AT campsites; the decision as to whether you "deserve" one is up to you. Aside from the three backpackers-only campgrounds (see page 91), people are prohibited from camping along the trail, except in designated shelters or near them. It should go without saying that you must be very careful to leave no trace when camping at these areas.

All shelters look pretty similar: a smallish, hewn-log

RATINGS

Beauty: ✩ ✩ ✩ ✩
Privacy: ✩ ✩ ✩
Spaciousness: ✩ ✩ ✩
Quiet: ✩ ✩ ✩
Security: ✩ ✩ ✩
Cleanliness: ✩ ✩ ✩

structure that appears faintly British. There are six primitive shelters along the Maryland portion of the AT. From north to south, they are: Devils Racecourse (0.2 miles from Pen Mar, near the Pennsylvania border), Ensign Cowall, Pine Knob, Rocky Run, Crampton Gap, and Ed Garvey, which is 3.5 miles north of the C&O Canal and the Potomac River beyond.

Because the overnight parking area just off US Route 40 and adjacent to I-70 is easy to get to and is the Maryland AT's almost mid-point, I'll operate under the assumption that all trips to the shelters begin from there. The closest shelter site by far is Pine Knob, which sits just 0.5 miles to the north; to reach the shelter, go west 0.1 mile from the AT on the blue-blazed trail.

Those wishing to pitch a tent at Pine Knob might find it a bit disappointing. It's often served as a partying spot, and it shows, with discarded beer cans and the like. That said, there is a lot of cleared space, so making do isn't so tough. The biggest downfall of this shelter is that you can hear I-70 in the distance. But its location provides some major

KEY INFORMATION

ADDRESS:	South Mountain State Park
	c/o Greenbrier State Park
	21843 National Pike
	Boonsboro, MD 21713
	(301) 791-4767
	Appalachian National Scenic Trail NPS Park Office
	Harpers Ferry Center
	Harpers Ferry, WV 25425
	(304) 535-6331
OPERATED BY:	South Mountain State Park is operated by the Maryland Department of Natural Resources; the Appalachian Trail is operated by the National Park Service and a consortium of local hiking and conservation organizations.
OPEN:	All year
SITES:	Shelters hold 4–10 people; each site allows for 5–10 tent sites
EACH SITE HAS:	Picnic table, fire ring, privy
ASSIGNMENT:	First come, first served
REGISTRATION:	None
FACILITIES:	Toilet (some have spring water)
PARKING:	None
FEE:	None
RESTRICTIONS:	*Pets:* Permitted on a leash
	Quiet Hours: Officially none
	Visitors: The Appalachian Trail Conservancy suggests hiking and camping in groups no larger than 10 people.
	Fires: In fire rings
	Alcohol: Not permitted
	Stay Limit: Practice and hikers' etiquette dictates short stays of 1–2 days during warmer months when demand is highest.
	Other: Allow thru-hikers first use of shelters

pluses: both Greenbrier State Park (see page 63) and George Washington State Park are nearby. The biggest nearby attraction is the short hike to Annapolis Rock, a beautiful perch that allows great vistas.

Continuing north: Ensign Cowall (replacing what AT old-timers would remember as the Hemlock Hill shelter) is 8.2 miles from Pine Knob. Ensign Cowall is an attractive structure, with a pitched wood roof and some very handsome triangular windows. It feels new and has some level ground nearby to pitch a tent.

The last shelter in this direction is Devils Racecourse, another 5 miles north. The tin roof on the Devils Racecourse is quite a step down from Ensign Cowall. Generally, the Devils Racecourse shelter isn't known as one of the AT's best. It's a bit run-down, and it requires a steep hike on loose rock of almost half a mile to reach it. If you're carrying lots of gear, it can be tough. Additionally, it's well known as a hangout and party spot for local kids looking for a place to drink. It's not unusual to see a pile of beer bottles or cans nearby. The upside is that the camping area is situated next to a clear and clean spring. Whether or not you choose to pitch your tent here, do make sure to visit the shelter's namesake: the Devil's Racecourse, a boulder field situated between rows of mature trees. If the haul from the Route 40/I-70 parking area is too far, you can reach this portion of the trail from Route 491 in Cascade and find overnight parking 5 miles north of the shelter, at the Pen Mar County Park.

If you're heading south from the Route 40/I-70 parking area, the first shelter along the route is Rocky Run, which is 6.9 miles south. (To reach the shelter, go west for 0.2 miles on the blue-blazed trail.) Rocky Run is one of my favorites; the setting is pristine, there's lots of space to camp (for level ground, head up the hill from the shelter to the fire pit), and a pipe sends clear, delicious spring water rushing out of the rocky hill. There's even a nicely constructed wooden swing near the shelter.

Crampton Gap is next, 5 miles from Rocky Run. AT thru-hikers often find Crampton Gap a pleasure—in recent years, it's been spiffed up with a new outhouse, a new deck with furniture, and a new fire ring. The downside is the rocky terrain—clearing a space for your tent takes a bit of maneuvering. Another access option for Crampton Gap is the overnight parking area at the Civil War Correspondents' Memorial on Gapland Road (MD Route 572), 1 mile west of Burkittsville.

Last is Ed Garvey, 4.1 miles from Crampton Gap. Ed Garvey is beautifully constructed. Upon approach, it looks more like a ski lodge than a primitive camping shelter. Picnic tables and massive crisscrossed logs make it an attractive place. Additionally, there's plenty of space for a tent, both right next to the shelter and on the little trails next to it. Ed Garvey allows easy access to Weverton Cliffs, which gives great views over the Potomac River and Harpers Ferry beyond.

MAP

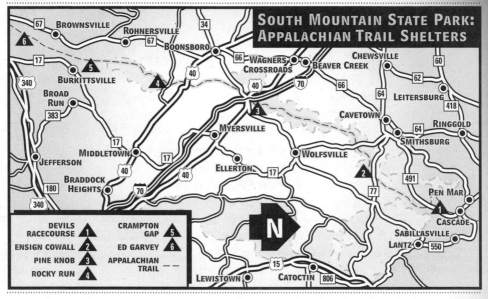

SOUTH MOUNTAIN STATE PARK: APPALACHIAN TRAIL SHELTERS

DEVILS RACECOURSE ▲1	CRAMPTON GAP ▲5
ENSIGN COWALL ▲2	ED GARVEY ▲6
PINE KNOB ▲3	APPALACHIAN TRAIL - - -
ROCKY RUN ▲4	

GETTING THERE

From I-70 East: Take Exit 42, MD Route 17. Bear right onto Route 17 North. Turn left onto US Route 40 West and follow for just over 3 miles to the parking area before I-70. From I-70 West: Take Exit 35 (MD Route 66). Bear right onto MD Route 66. Turn left onto US Route 40 East. Follow for 2.5 miles to the parking area on the right.

GPS COORDINATES

UTM Zone (NAD27) 18S
Easting 276217
Northing 4379490

27
SOUTH MOUNTAIN STATE PARK: APPALACHIAN TRAIL BACKPACKERS' CAMPGROUNDS (ANNAPOLIS ROCK, DAHLGREN, POGO)

For AT thru-hikers, Dahlgren is a veritable Shangri-La.

SOUTH MOUNTAIN STATE PARK runs some 8,039 acres, following the ridge of South Mountain from Pen Mar, just south of the Pennsylvania border, to Weverton, just north of the Potomac River; the total park acreage is over 10,000 and includes the South Mountain State Battlefield, site of the September 1862 Civil War battle. The park provides year-round access to the Appalachian Trail. The trail itself, as many know, goes more than 2,000 miles from Maine to Georgia. Maryland's AT portion is 41 miles, running along the borders of Washington and Frederick Counties.

There are three backpackers' campgrounds along the Maryland section of the AT: Dahlgren (something of a legend for AT thru-hikers), Pogo, and the newest, Annapolis Rock. Using the Maryland AT (roughly) mid-point overnight parking area off US 40, Pogo is 4 miles north, Annapolis Rock is 2.2 miles north, and Dahlgren is 5.2 miles south. The ratings below represent averages for the three sites and will vary according to season; for instance, "privacy" and "quiet" will skyrocket in winter and plummet in summer.

Pogo Campground is really one big area cleared for roughly a dozen or so tents. The ground is pretty level, so there's no big problem setting up. A spring issues cold, clear water just a few feet from the trail. Often, privies at such primitive campgrounds like Pogo are situated between sites. Wisely, this one is up the hill, so if it gets to emanate a bad smell, you should be far enough that it won't bother you.

Closer to the parking area is Annapolis Rock. The good news here is that the campsites are new, the result of a concerted effort from the Maryland Department of Natural Resources, the AT Conference, and conservationists from the Virginia Polytechnic Institute. In 2004, the U.S. Department of the Interior

RATINGS

Beauty: ✿ ✿ ✿ ✿
Privacy: ✿ ✿ ✿
Spaciousness: ✿ ✿ ✿
Quiet: ✿ ✿ ✿
Security: ✿ ✿ ✿
Cleanliness: ✿ ✿ ✿ ✿

recognized the campground and trail with admission to the National Recreation Trails System. Those who've camped at Annapolis Rock in the past have known some real ambivalence about the experience. For one, its namesake attraction is obvious: an outstanding perch above beautiful rolling and forested mountains. Waking up with the sun in such a place is an extraordinary way to start a day (and watching it set later that day is magical). But the refrain in describing Annapolis Rock over the years has been that it's "loved to death." Legions of campers have stripped the area of wood for fires, the soil has been made barren by a multitude of fires, and trash has collected.

In 2002, work crews began constructing campsites in a thickly vegetated area, away from the rock cliff, and the following spring began re-vegetating the denuded area. The new campsite is great. It has 14 individual sites that hold up to 75 campers, it has two privies, and it hosts a caretaker to minimize harmful impact practices. The sites are built into the hillside to prevent erosion, and they are comparatively private as a result.

KEY INFORMATION

ADDRESS:	South Mountain State Park
	c/o Greenbrier State Park
	21843 National Pike
	Boonsboro, MD 21713
	(301) 791-4767
	Appalachian National Scenic Trail NPS Park Office
	Harpers Ferry Center
	Harpers Ferry, WV 25425
	(304) 535-6331
OPERATED BY:	South Mountain State Park is operated by the Maryland Department of Natural Resources; the Appalachian Trail is operated by the National Park Service and a consortium of local hiking and conservation organizations.
OPEN:	All year
SITES:	35 (14 at Annapolis Rock, 5 at Dahlgren, 16 at Pogo)
EACH SITE HAS:	Picnic table, fire ring (at Pogo and Dahlgren), privy, water
ASSIGNMENT:	First come, first served
REGISTRATION:	None
FACILITIES:	Showers at Dahlgren; water shut off March to December
PARKING:	None
FEE:	None
RESTRICTIONS:	*Pets:* Permitted on a leash
	Quiet Hours: Officially none, but loud music or noises are discouraged
	Visitors: The Appalachian Trail Conservancy suggests hiking and camping in groups no larger than 10 people. Larger groups will be directed away from Annapolis Rock.
	Fires: In fire rings only (no fires at Annapolis Rock)
	Alcohol: Not permitted
	Stay Limit: Practice and hikers' etiquette dictates short stays of 1–2 days during warmer months, when demand is highest.
	Other: Limit visits on weekends, holidays, and during peak fall foliage

MAP

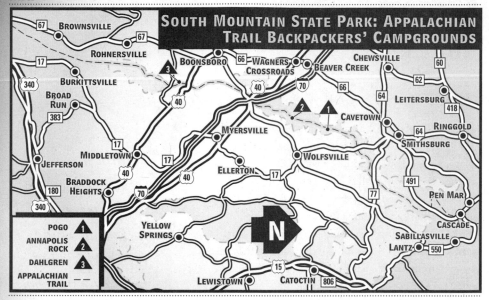

SOUTH MOUNTAIN STATE PARK: APPALACHIAN TRAIL BACKPACKERS' CAMPGROUNDS

POGO 1
ANNAPOLIS ROCK 2
DAHLGREN 3
APPALACHIAN TRAIL – –

GETTING THERE

From the East: On I-70, take Exit 42, MD Route 17. Bear right onto Route 17 North. Turn left onto US Route 40 West and follow it for just over 3 miles to the parking area before I-70.

From the West: On I-70, take Exit 35, MD Route 66. Bear right onto Route 66. Turn left onto US Route 40 East. Follow for 2.5 miles to the parking area on the right.

GPS COORDINATES

UTM Zone (NAD27) 18S
Easting 276217
Northing 4379490

The only campground south of the parking area, Dahlgren Backpackers Campground, is diminutive, with only five tent pads, each with a picnic table and a grill. However, there is a lot of cleared space between the trees and the tent pads, enough for dozens more tents, which is the usual practice. For AT thru-hikers, Dahlgren is a veritable Shangri-La. There's one reason for this: free hot showers (in season), the only of their kind for some 2,000 miles of the AT. However, the hot water is shut off during the off-season, December to March. Two miles north of Dahlgren is Washington Monument State Park, home of the country's first monument to our first president, erected in 1827.

One of the nice things about these three campsites is that they sit within 10 miles of each other. You can easily camp at each in successive nights without having to haul gear very far; the myriad side trails and numerous attractions in the area make this portion of the AT a truly wonderful place to hike and camp.

28
SWALLOW FALLS STATE PARK

LIKE NATURE? Swallow Falls State Park is the ticket. Within this relatively small park (257 acres), you'll find three waterfalls (including Muddy Creek Falls, Maryland's tallest single-drop waterfall), the Youghiogheny Wild and Scenic River, and the oldest white pine and eastern hemlock in the state, some trees approaching 400 years old. The park's name derives from the cliff swallows that used to nest on the rock pillar below the upper Swallow Falls. Long before it became a park the area was drawing admirers. Some of the legends of American entrepreneurship (Ford, Firestone, and Edison, among them) camped along the falls, hoping for inspiration. Though your trip here won't be nearly as rugged, you can draw inspiration just the same within some spectacular scenery.

The trail network near and around the falls can get crowded during the summer, but hiking along here is a treat nonetheless. If you want more privacy (and a rugged hike), head for the 5-mile trail to Herrington Manor Park to the south along a defunct tram road used for logging in the 1800s. The trail between the two parks takes in streams and hardwood forests home of black bears, among other woodland creatures.

There's the fishing in the Youghiogheny, too. Each year, the river is stocked with rainbow and brown trout. Native fish species include rock and smallmouth bass, chub, and white and northern hog sucker.

The majority of visitors to Swallow Falls will be day-trippers taking advantage of the easy trails running through hemlock forests and along the Youghiogheny River, where one can take in Muddy Creek, Upper Swallow, Lower Swallow, and Tolliver Falls. As a result, the park can get quite crowded during the day, but the campsite–because it is reached by heading left when everyone else goes right–feels relatively secluded

> *Within this relatively small park, you'll find three waterfalls, including Muddy Creek Falls, Maryland's tallest single-drop waterfall.*

RATINGS

Beauty: ☆ ☆ ☆ ☆ ☆
Privacy: ☆ ☆ ☆
Spaciousness: ☆ ☆
Quiet: ☆ ☆ ☆
Security: ☆ ☆ ☆ ☆ ☆
Cleanliness: ☆ ☆ ☆ ☆ ☆

and peaceful. Your two camping choices are the Garrett Loop and the Tolliver Loop, which come after the youth group area. Even if you're not staying in the youth group area, it is here where you can access the 5-mile trail to Herrington Manor Park.

First up is Garrett Loop, with sites 1 to 5, 7, 33, 35, 37, 39, and 40 to 64. The ones on the outside of the loops (odd-numbered) are usually preferable because they afford slightly more privacy. Sites 43 and 45 are the most isolated. Tent-only sites in this loop are 33, 46, 49, and 50; of these, site 49 is my favorite, as it has a bit of a drop-off on each side. Site 33 sits very near the loop's electric sites (40, 42, and 42a), but it's also within a nice little group of pines. The largest sites in the Garrett Loop are 2, 5, 7, and 35, all of them 30 feet. All others in the Garrett Loop range from 12 to 27 feet. Two wheelchair-accessible sites, 4 and 60, are also available.

Tolliver Loop contains sites 6, 8, 9 to 32, 34, 36, and 38. Tolliver sits beyond Garrett and so sees a bit less car traffic. It also has fewer sites total, which is also an advantage. Sites 30, 32, and 34 are in a nice spot on the outer lower edge, across from the path to the

KEY INFORMATION

ADDRESS:	Swallow Falls State Park
	c/o Herrington Manor State Park
	222 Herrington Lane
	Oakland, MD 21550
	(301) 387-6938
OPERATED BY:	Maryland Department of Natural Resources
OPEN:	Late May–mid-October for both loops; Garrett Loop opens in mid-April and stays open until mid-December
SITES:	65
EACH SITE HAS:	Fire ring, picnic table, lantern post, tent pad
ASSIGNMENT:	Reservations recommended in summer; first come, first served in both loops during May and September–October and in Garrett Loop mid-April–May and October–mid-December
REGISTRATION:	(888) 432-2267 or online at http://reservations.dnr.state.md.us
FACILITIES:	Picnic area, pavilion, playground, bathhouse
PARKING:	Max. 2 vehicles per site
FEE:	$25/night, $35/night electric, water, and sewer; day-use service charge: Memorial Day–Labor Day, $2/person; out-of-state residents add $1 to service charges
RESTRICTIONS:	*Pets:* Allowed in the campground but not permitted in the day-use area from the Saturday before Memorial Day–Labor Day
	Quiet Hours: 11 p.m.–7 a.m.
	Visitors: Max. 6 people at each site
	Fires: In fire ring only
	Alcohol: Must remain at the site
	Stay Limit: 2 weeks
	Other: 2-night minimum stay for weekends, 3-night for holiday weekends. Check-out is 3 p.m., and check-in must be done before 11 p.m. Mid-October–December is primitive camping. This is bear country; take proper precautions.

MAP

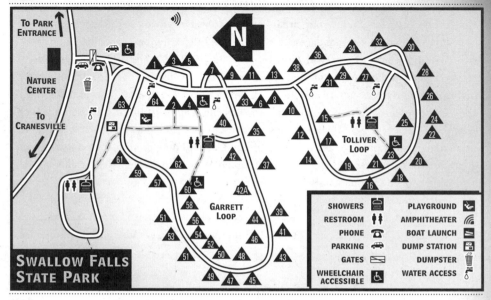

SWALLOW FALLS
STATE PARK

bathhouse. Sites 8, 10, 12, 19, 21, 23, and 33 are tent-only. If you require lots of room, several sites—9, 11, 13, 15, and 27—are significantly larger than the others. Site 6, at 36 feet, is the largest in all of Swallow Falls.

Overall, there isn't too much space separating these relatively small sites, but they are nicely wooded and pleasant nonetheless. Because of the limited number of sites, the campground doesn't feel very packed. My preference is for the Tolliver Loop, as most sites sit within pine and hemlock copses, which are exceedingly pleasant.

GETTING THERE

Take I-68 to exit 14, MD Route 219 South. Go 20 miles to Mayhew Inn Road and turn right. At the stop sign at the end of the road, turn left onto Oakland Sang Run Road. Take the first right onto Swallow Falls Road.

GPS COORDINATES

UTM Zone (NAD27) 17S
Easting 632975
Northing 4373181

> *After its spectacular Class IV–V rapids in Maryland, the Youghiogheny River is dammed, producing the recreational haven of Youghiogheny River Lake.*

MOST PEOPLE IN THE TRI-STATE area (Maryland–Pennsylvania–West Virginia) regard Youghiogheny River Lake as a Pennsylvania possession. Indeed, though the lake straddles the Mason–Dixon Line, the majority of it lies in Pennsylvania. Furthermore, the majority of whitewater rafting trips down the Youghiogheny commence from Pennsylvania locations: Ohiopyle and Confluence, to be precise (though real whitewater aficionados head for the Upper Yough, from Sang Run to Friendsville, in Maryland).

The river flows northward and, after its spectacular Class IV-V rapids in Maryland, it's dammed, producing the recreational haven of Youghiogheny River Lake. The U.S. Army Corps of Engineers maintains three campsites along the lake; two of them (Outflow and Tub Run) sit in Pennsylvania. They are the larger two of the three and are worth a visit. (You can contact Outflow and Tub Run by calling (877) 444-6777, or online at **www.reserveusa.com.**) Here I'll concentrate solely on Youghiogheny River Lake's only Maryland campsite: Mill Run.

Despite containing a boat launch for the lake, the campground feels nicely isolated, partly due to the fact that it sits in a sparsely populated area of the state. Additionally, Mill Run Campground sits in a woodsy copse adjoining the Mill Run, a tributary of the Youghiogheny. Because the other two campgrounds on the lake are significantly larger and more popular, Mill Run feels like paradise found. This is not to say that you shouldn't expect company during the day, especially in summer.

If you're a boater, take advantage of what is widely considered the best boating and waterskiing lake anywhere near. If you've brought along the fishing pole, angle for walleye, bass, and trout. And, of course, there's always the whitewater rafting. After

RATINGS

Beauty: ✪ ✪ ✪ ✪ ✪
Privacy: ✪ ✪
Quiet: ✪ ✪ ✪ ✪
Spaciousness: ✪ ✪ ✪
Security: ✪ ✪ ✪ ✪ ✪
Cleanliness: ✪ ✪ ✪ ✪

West Virginia's Gauley River, the Yough is arguably the East's best whitewater rafting locale.

Beyond the lake itself, recreational activities abound to the south. The Youghiogheny Scenic and Wild River was named as such in 1976, becoming Maryland's first river with such a designation. A 21-mile stretch from Friendsville to Oakland remains protected and thrives as a beautiful and clean river even though it retains its popularity as a whitewater rafting hotspot. (For recreational opportunities on the Youghiogheny Scenic and Wild River, contact the Maryland State Forest and Park Service, c/o Deep Creek Lake Recreation Area, 898 State Park Road, Swanton, MD 21561; (301) 387-5563). As for the campground itself, it is a bit rustic, to put it nicely. Scoffers will call it run down. I would call it a great place to stay for cheap that offers access to the lake. Some of the sites (15 to 18) are spitting distance from the boat ramp, with site 18 being the closest. The first few sites (1 to 8) are near the campground entrance and are not terribly special. They sit literally right next to one another. But the farther you move to the right, the more private the sites get, with site 11 being the best in terms of privacy. My favorite sites in the campground are those down the hill across from the camp host, numbered 23 to 30. The most private

KEY INFORMATION

ADDRESS:	Contact: 497 Flanigan Road
	Confluence, PA 15424-1902
	(814) 395-3242
	Physical: Mill Run Recreation Area
	Friendsville, MD 21531
OPERATED BY:	U.S. Army Corps of Engineers
OPEN:	All year (reduced facilities mid-September–April)
SITES:	30
EACH SITE HAS:	Table and fire ring
ASSIGNMENT:	First-come, first served
REGISTRATION:	Self-registration May–mid-September; no registration required otherwise
FACILITIES:	Restrooms (no showers), playground, dump station, drinking water, phone, swimming beach, boat launch
PARKING:	Vehicles not allowed on grass; multiple units allowed at each campsite so long as they fit within the boundaries of the site
FEE:	When self-registration is in effect: $12/night, $15/night electric, $26/night electric, water, and sewer. Hike and bike, $4. Pay by check to Army Corps of Engineers, Pittsburgh; free mid-September–end of April
RESTRICTIONS:	*Pets:* Must be leashed or caged
	Quiet Hours: 10 p.m.–6 a.m.
	Visitors: Max. 6 people per site; guests must leave by 10 p.m.
	Fires: In fire rings
	Alcohol: Not permitted
	Stay Limit: 2-week limit within 30 days
	Other: Check-out 4 p.m.

MAP

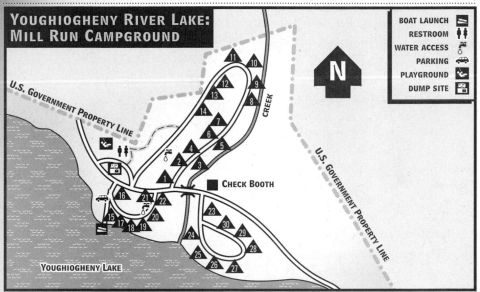

YOUGHIOGHENY RIVER LAKE: MILL RUN CAMPGROUND

BOAT LAUNCH
RESTROOM
WATER ACCESS
PARKING
PLAYGROUND
DUMP SITE

N

U.S. GOVERNMENT PROPERTY LINE

CREEK

U.S. GOVERNMENT PROPERTY LINE

CHECK BOOTH

YOUGHIOGHENY LAKE

GETTING THERE

Take I-68 to Exit 4, MD Route 53 North, Friendsville-Addison Road. Go through Friendsville and look for the signs to Mill Run to the left.

ones are 26 and 27, as they sit on the farthest edge of the campground.

Remember, if you want to be in the center of all the action around Yough River Lake, head for the Pennsylvania campsites. (From Mill Run, if you continue up Friendsville-Addison Road and then go left at Addison, you'll get to the main recreation areas of the lake.) Mill Run is a bit away from it all, but this can be a good thing.

GPS COORDINATES

UTM Zone (NAD27) 17S
Easting 638513
Northing 4397498

CENTRAL MARYLAND

30
LOUISE F. COSCA REGIONAL PARK

COSCA REGIONAL PARK began life in 1967 as Clinton Regional Park, Prince George's County's first regional park. A few years after its inception, its name was changed to honor the former Park and Planning Commissioner who saw it to its fruition. If she were around today, Ms. Cosca would no doubt be unhappy about the choc-a-bloc development just down Thrift Road from the park. But the park itself feels that much more an oasis as a result.

Admittedly, I didn't have very high hopes upon my first visit to Cosca. The park sits in Clinton, a populated D.C. suburb that no one would ever associate with good camping. But what a pleasant surprise awaited me. First, the park itself is very much a family affair, with recreation galore: ball fields, a tennis bubble, picnic areas, a lake and boathouse, a nature center, and the Cosca Cannonball, a miniature train which offers rides for the not-so-princely sum of 75 cents.

At 600 acres, the park is a decent size and offers more than 5 miles of trails for hiking or horseback riding. At the lake, folks can fish year-round and boat during the warmer months. The lake is stocked with bass, bluegill, catfish, and trout. The Clearwater Nature Center is truly a community affair, offering loads of nature programs geared toward kids and adults. There's an Outdoor Explorers Club for kids ages 5 to 7.

What's especially nice is that the campground is across the road from the major sites listed above. As a result, it feels nicely secluded, but hiking trails link you easily to the rest of the park. The sites are wooded,

> *Cosca Regional Park is very much a family affair, with recreation galore.*

RATINGS

Beauty: ✩ ✩ ✩
Privacy: ✩ ✩ ✩ ✩
Spaciousness: ✩ ✩ ✩
Quiet: ✩ ✩ ✩
Security: ✩ ✩ ✩ ✩
Cleanliness: ✩ ✩ ✩ ✩

ADDRESS: Cosca Regional Park
11000 Thrift Road
Clinton, MD 20735
(301) 868-1397

OPERATED BY: Maryland National
Capital Park
and Planning
Commission

OPEN: All year

SITES: 25 (including
2 group sites)

EACH SITE HAS: Picnic table, fire
ring, tent pad

ASSIGNMENT: First come, first
served

REGISTRATION: At the park office

FACILITIES: Picnic areas and
shelters, tennis
courts, ball fields,
boathouse, play-
grounds, comfort
stations

PARKING: On paved areas only

FEE: Prince George's and
Montgomery County
residents: $15/night,
$18/night electric;
nonresidents,
$20 and $23,
respectively

RESTRICTIONS: *Pets:* On a leash
Quiet Hours: 10 p.m.–
7 a.m.
Visitors: No policy
Fires: In fire rings
only
Alcohol: Not allowed
Stay Limit: 2 weeks
Other: Max. 1 camp-
ing unit per site

with generally 50 feet or so between them. There's a picnic area, a playground, and a bathhouse in the camping area, and everything is kept well maintained and clean. To get a site, head to the campground, pick whichever available one you like, then go to the park office and pay your fee. Be sure to avoid sites 9, 11, and, to a lesser extent, 12; you can see residential houses through the trees behind these sites—the best way to spoil the illusion of sleeping out in nature. Sites 8 and 9 are reserved for groups of 15 to 30 people.

Site 13 is nice, as it sits by itself. Site 14 is also good, and 1 to 8 are decent. Site 15 has the drawback of not being very level. Sites 16 to 22 seem to be the best: 16 has two picnic tables and pump water and is very spacious, 17 is nicely secluded, 18 is big, and 19 is my favorite. For this site, you pull into the parking area, and the tent site is off to the left another ten yards or so deeper in the woods. Sites 21 and 22 have a similar setup.

MAP

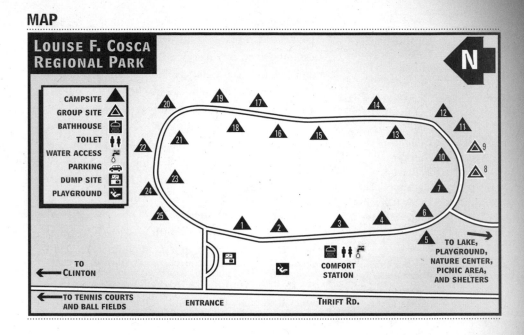

N

CAMPSITE
GROUP SITE
BATHHOUSE
TOILET
WATER ACCESS
PARKING
DUMP SITE
PLAYGROUND

TO LAKE,
PLAYGROUND,
NATURE CENTER,
PICNIC AREA,
AND SHELTERS

COMFORT
STATION

TO
CLINTON

TO TENNIS COURTS
AND BALL FIELDS

ENTRANCE

THRIFT RD.

GETTING THERE

Take I-495 to Exit 7A South (Branch Avenue/MD Route 5) toward Waldorf. Make a right onto Woodyard Road. Turn left onto Brandywine Road. Make a right onto Thrift Road.

GPS COORDINATES

UTM Zone (NAD27) 18S
Easting 334148
Northing 4289412

31
CEDARVILLE
STATE FOREST

> *Spring is a fantastic time to come to Cedarville, as the wildflowers that dot the swamplands explode in color.*

IT PAINS ME NOW, but I grew up within an hour of Cedarville State Forest (3,510 acres) and never knew of its existence until recently, now that I live much farther away. But better late then never; it's a great place.

The Piscataway Indians knew this, choosing the area around Cedarville Forest as their winter camping ground. They were well adapted to the ecology of the area, which is adjacent to the largest freshwater swamp in the state, Zekiah Swamp, which drains into the Wicomico River, some 20 miles away. The park contains the Cedarville Bog, at the swamp headwaters, allowing for an environment Marylanders don't see so much of, as the atmosphere conjures something closer to the Southeast. Correspondingly, insect-eating plants, a relative rarity in Maryland, flourish here. Diamond-back terrapins, a state mascot, live within the swamp areas and its tributaries. Bald eagles also nest here. With 19 miles of trails in the forest, a hiker can cover them all in a few days and take in the forest's wonderful ecological treasures. If all the forest and swampland isn't enough, there's also the four-acre Cedarville Pond, stocked with bass, bluegill, catfish, and sunfish (a Maryland nontidal sportfishing license is required). The pond area, accessible from the Green and Brown Trails down the forest road and over Zekiah Swamp Run, is the best place to see the swamp environment. A managed forest conservation area hosts some 50 different tree species.

Spring is a fantastic time to come here, as the wildflowers that dot the swamplands explode in color. An abundance of wildlife thrives in the managed forest, while the swamp waters attract loads of beaver and birds.

Cedarville State Forest has 27 sites in one loop, past the youth group camping area. Of the 27 sites, 12

RATINGS

Beauty: ✪ ✪ ✪ ✪
Privacy: ✪ ✪ ✪ ✪
Spaciousness: ✪ ✪ ✪
Quiet: ✪ ✪ ✪ ✪
Security: ✪ ✪ ✪ ✪ ✪
Cleanliness: ✪ ✪ ✪ ✪ ✪

are walk-in (sites 1, 6, 7, 13, 14, 16, 17, 18, 20, 22, 24, and 26). Site 2 is reserved for the camp host. The rest are reservable. Sites 4, 6, 8, 10, 12, 14, 16, 18, 20, 22, and 24 are electric. All these sit on the internal section of the loop; what this means is that you'll want to shoot for the external sites. Among them, the sites that sit farthest from the electric (RV) sites are 7, 1, 2, 3, 26, and 27. The only bathhouse sits in the middle of the loop. Firewood can be purchased at the campground (eight pieces for $2). There's also spring water available.

The campsites are very well shaded and spaced. There's often 100 feet or more between sites. Many sites sit right across the road from one another (as opposed to staggered) and thus don't offer oodles of privacy. The camping area is very small, and it's easy to feel close to your neighbors. The sites on the outside of the loop seem to be the better ones, as they're slightly more private. Of these, I think that 17, 19, and 21 are the nicest. Sites 1 and 3 are also nice—there's lots of space around them. For walk-in, just pick a spot marked available and drop your money in the envelope at the bulletin board.

KEY INFORMATION

ADDRESS: Southern Maryland Recreational Complex Cedarville State Forest 10201 Bee Oak Road Brandywine, MD 20613 (301) 888-1410

OPERATED BY: Maryland Department of Natural Resources

OPEN: End of April–end of October

SITES: 27

EACH SITE HAS: Parking pad, picnic table, fire ring

ASSIGNMENT: Walk-in and reservable

REGISTRATION: (888) 432-CAMP (2267) or online at http://reservations .dnr.state.md.us

FACILITIES: Bathhouse, pavilion, dump station

PARKING: 2 vehicles per site

FEE: $20/night, $25/night electric

RESTRICTIONS: *Pets:* Permitted
Quiet Hours: 11 p.m.–7 a.m.
Visitors: Max. 6 people, 2 tents
Fires: In fire rings
Alcohol: Restricted to sites
Stay Limit: 2 weeks
Other: 2-day minimum required Memorial Day–Labor Day

MAP

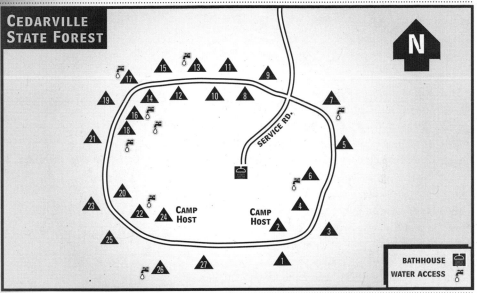

CEDARVILLE STATE FOREST

GETTING THERE

From I-495, take Exit 7A,
MD Route 5 South (Branch
Avenue) toward Waldorf. Follow Route 5 until it ends at
US Route 301 and follow it
south. Turn left at the stop
light onto Cedarville Road
(look for the state forest sign).
Turn right at Bee Oak Road.

GPS COORDINATES

UTM Zone (NAD27) 18S
Easting 342236
Northing 4279409

SITUATED ON A PENINSULA BETWEEN the Chesapeake Bay and the Elk River, Elk Neck State Park contains a wealth of beauty (though no elk), encapsulated within a real diversity in topography, including beaches, marshes, and forests. Despite this, even on busy weekends, there's almost always a spot to stay, so you can feel comfortable making a last-minute decision to go and get a walk-in site.

Elk Neck remains a perfect place for families wishing to camp, drawing folks from Baltimore, Philadelphia, and Delaware. Expect crowds and not much privacy. Still, it's difficult to spend a few days at Elk Neck and not have a pleasant experience. Fishing, birding, hiking, boating, and swimming are popular activities.

Several friends of mine who wouldn't have considered camping there before find it perfect now that they have children. One of the consistent remarks among visitors is how amazingly clean this park manages to remain. Considering the heavy usage, it's a real testament to the staff. While it may be difficult to achieve total privacy at a popular park like Elk Neck, essentially every loop sits near a hiking trail or the water, so it's not difficult to escape, and the scenery never fails to impress.

Turkey Point Road (MD Route 272) is the main road that splits the park and ends at the parking area for the popular Blue Trail with its main attraction, the Turkey Point Lighthouse. Highest of the Chesapeake Bay's 74 lighthouses, it was built in 1833. But before you get there, you'll turn left on Campground Access Road. From there, you can reach any of Elk Neck's 12 camping loops (though some are for youth groups and some contain cabins). After passing the registration booth, if you take the first right you'll come first to the North East Loop, which contains 31 sites, all of them with full hookups for RVs; North East also allows leashed pets.

Pass North East and you'll eventually come to five more loops. First up to the right are the Wye Loop and the Susquehanna Loop. Wye contains sites 32 to 61,

> *One of the consistent remarks among visitors is how amazingly clean this park manages to remain.*

RATINGS

Beauty: ☆ ☆ ☆ ☆
Privacy: ☆ ☆
Spaciousness: ☆ ☆
Quiet: ☆ ☆ ☆
Security: ☆ ☆ ☆ ☆ ☆
Cleanliness: ☆ ☆ ☆ ☆ ☆

Susquehanna has sites 62 to 75. Pets, so long as they are leashed, are allowed in both loops. One thing that should be noted here, though it may seem counterintuitive: Several park rangers have suggested to me that the pet loops are among the nicest in the park, because the others cater to RVs and can get much louder. So don't be too quick to dismiss the pet loops if you don't have a dog. If barking doggies are not your bag, however, continue on to the end of the road, where you'll run into the three remaining loops: Choptank to the left, Elk to the right, and Miles straight ahead.

Choptank (sites 91 to 120) sits closest to the White Trail, an interpretive foliage trail across from the large camp store. The entrance to Elk Loop (sites 122 to 151) is close to a playground (especially sites 122 to 124), but its southern edge (sites 136 to 139) is near Stony Point and Rogues Harbor and allows easy access for a vigorous trek through forest, beach, and marsh on the Orange Trail.

Last in this bunch is the Miles Loop (sites 152 to 181), closest of all to Stony Point and its attendant views over the mighty Elk River. If you do stay in Miles Loop, try to snag sites 162, 163, or 165, as they are nearest the water.

Here's something of a secret: Along the camp road to these three loops is St. Martin's Loop, a tent section that does not show up on all park maps. Between Susquehanna and Elk, St. Martin's 15 sites (76 to 90) tend not to fill up as quickly as the more prominent sites. You're not far from several other loops, but in this part of the park that's your best bet for privacy. Also, St. Martin sits close to the wonderful Orange Trail.

KEY INFORMATION

ADDRESS: Elk Neck State Park
4395 Turkey Point Road
North East, MD 21901
(410) 287-5333; Park-ElkNeck@dnr.state.md.us

OPERATED BY: Maryland Department of Natural Resources

OPEN: All year in Chester and North East Loops; late March–September in Elk Loop; late March–October in Wye and Miles loops; mid April–early September in Bohemia, Susquehanna, and Choptank loops

SITES: 278

EACH SITE HAS: Fire ring, picnic table, tent pad

ASSIGNMENT: Reservable and walk-in

REGISTRATION: (888) 432-CAMP, online at http://reservations/dnr.state.md.us, or walk-in at the Ranger Station on Campground Access Road

FACILITIES: Boat launch, cabins, camp store, dump station, playground, shelters, swimming beach, visitor center

PARKING: 2 vehicles per site

FEE: $25/night, $30/night electric, $35 water and sewer; day-use fee: April–October, weekdays $3/vehicle, weekends and holidays $3/person; boat launch, $10/vehicle; out-of-state residents add $1 to all charges. Seniors (62+) camp half price, Sunday–Thursday

RESTRICTIONS: *Pets:* Leashed pets are allowed in North East, Wye, and Susquehanna loops
Quiet Hours: 11 p.m.–7 a.m.
Visitors: 6 people, 2 tents per site ($3 per person over maximum)
Fires: In fire rings
Alcohol: Allowed
Stay Limit: 2 weeks

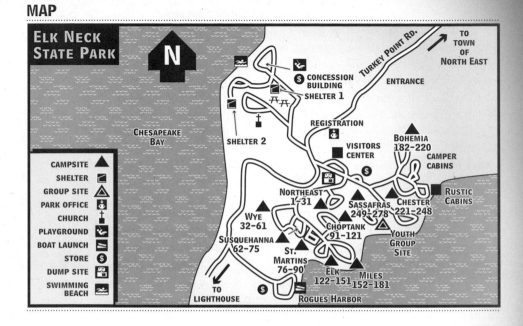

ELK NECK
STATE PARK

N

TO
TOWN
OF
NORTH EAST

TURKEY POINT RD.

CONCESSION
BUILDING
SHELTER 1

ENTRANCE

CHESAPEAKE
BAY

SHELTER 2

REGISTRATION

VISITORS
CENTER

BOHEMIA
182–220

CAMPER
CABINS

CAMPSITE
SHELTER
GROUP SITE
PARK OFFICE
CHURCH
PLAYGROUND
BOAT LAUNCH
STORE
DUMP SITE
SWIMMING
BEACH

NORTHEAST
1–31

SASSAFRAS
249–278

CHESTER
221–248

RUSTIC
CABINS

WYE
32–61

CHOPTANK
91–121

YOUTH
GROUP
SITE

SUSQUEHANNA
62–75

ST.
MARTINS
76–90

ELK
122–151

MILES
152–181

TO
LIGHTHOUSE

ROGUES HARBOR

Your other option for camping is northeast of the loops described above. Take the same Campground Access Road, but this time pass the registration booth and keep going straight, past the playground and camp store (which has laundry, by the way). Then you can either go left for Chester and Bohemia loops or right for the Sassafras Loop. The youth group area sits beyond Sassafras at the end of the road.

Sassafras loop sits adjacent to an open field, which can be a pleasant way to camp, often overlooked by people who assume the more woods the better. Sites 249 to 257 all sit at the edge of the road, with the open field behind. The better sites are those farther out, 258 to 277.

Bohemia (sites 182 to 206 and 217 to 220) is a circular loop near the beach areas north of Thackeray Point and allows easy access to the Green Trail, which winds along marsh and small lakes. If you camp in Bohemia, definitely try to get Site 196, which is not just tent-only but also sits right up the hill from the water.

Lastly, Chester Loop (sites 221 to 248) feels most crowded, with the sites near one another in a series of little roads running between the loop ends. The best ones here, in my opinion, are sites 221, 222, and 233, as they sit on the outside of the loop and near only one other site.

GETTING THERE

Take I-95 from Baltimore to Exit 100 (MD Route 272 South) to North East. Elk Neck is 10 miles south of North East.

GPS COORDINATES

UTM Zone (NAD27) 18S
Easting 415332
Northing 4369813

> *In 2006, every state but two had a representative camper in Greenbelt.*

WHEN THE FEDERAL GOVERNMENT acquired land to build the Baltimore–Washington Parkway (Route 295) in 1950, Greenbelt Park (1,100 acres) was established as a sanctuary between the two big cities. It sits just 12 miles north of Washington and 23 miles south of Baltimore. Nowadays the corridor between Baltimore and Washington is highly developed. But Greenbelt Park remains a green sanctuary, albeit a very popular one. According to the National Park Service, some 350,000 people visit the park annually, 20,000 of whom stay to camp. The result is that you won't feel very alone or as if you're roughing it. A unique characteristic of Greenbelt Park is that it functions as an inexpensive lodging alternative for visitors to D.C.; especially during the summer tourist season, your camp neighbor may very well be from across the country, or even across the globe. In fact, every state but two (Wyoming and Alaska) had a representative camper in Greenbelt in 2006. This can make for some interesting conversation.

The park's proximity to the capital is its chief attraction, but if you already live here, it is still a fine place to spend a few days. Wildlife isn't terribly exotic in the park, but it's abundant (my favorite are the foxes). A good place to spot wildlife, as well as enjoy some towering forest, is on the park's 6-mile Perimeter Trail. Aside from weaving through a deciduous forest, it also takes in three different creeks along the way.

Many visitors see the fact that the park is surrounded by major traffic arteries as a chief turn-off. But if you live in either city and need a quick escape, you couldn't ask for a better, more convenient choice. Additionally, the traffic noise isn't too bad. In fact, when I camped here in summer, the sounds of cicadas during the day and crickets at night effectively masked traffic noise. Further, because there are no electrical

RATINGS

Beauty: ☆ ☆ ☆
Privacy: ☆ ☆ ☆
Spaciousness: ☆ ☆ ☆
Quiet: ☆ ☆ ☆
Security: ☆ ☆ ☆ ☆ ☆
Cleanliness: ☆ ☆ ☆ ☆ ☆

hookups at any of the campsites, you need not worry about RV electrical noise.

From Park Central Road, you'll access the four camping loops: A, B, C, and D. Skip A entirely, as it is reserved only for scouts. In terms of noise, the best bet is probably C, which sits the farthest from the major roads that hem the park, though the difference in traffic noise between this loop and the others is probably negligible. Adding to the allure of Loop C, however, is the fact that it is tent-only. Aside from this, most of the campsites in the park are very similar. The biggest difference between them lies in the sites that have long driveways for RVs. Overall, the campsites are very clean and well maintained.

All sites are wooded and nicely shaded but without much room between them. In some cases, it's barely ten feet from one campsite to the next. The most you'll ever find between sites is around 75 feet. Nevertheless, most sites do back up to thick woods, so while they all sit very close to the campground roads and neighbors, if you face your tent toward the back of the site, you'll give yourself the illusion of isolation.

I prefer Loop C because of its tent-only status. This fact alone makes the loop feel closest to camping in the woods. However, the sites offering the most privacy, I found, are in Loop D. Site 174 is small but away from other campsites (though close to the campground road and the bathhouse). Sites 138 to 143 are open, in the middle of the camp loop, ideal for stargazing. Sites on the outside of the loop, such as 147 and 149, tend to be the biggest and most private.

In Loop B, sites 79 and 71 are nice, but my favorite is Site 81, because it has a little parking area and the tent area is just up a little rise in deeper woods.

You're never too far from something at Greenbelt. Its proximity to the capital, its wooded sites, and its fine hiking trails are worth a visit.

KEY INFORMATION

ADDRESS: 6565 Greenbelt Rd. Greenbelt, MD 20770 (301) 344-3948

OPERATED BY: National Park Service

OPEN: All year

SITES: 174

EACH SITE HAS: Fire grate, picnic table

ASSIGNMENT: Reservable Memorial Day–Labor Day; first come, first served otherwise. If the office is closed, self-register at the bulletin board just beyond the park office.

REGISTRATION: (877) 444-6777, online at www .recreation.gov, or at Park Ranger Station open daily from 8 a.m.– 3:45 p.m.

FACILITIES: Restrooms, picnic tables, water, fireplaces, utility sinks, dump station

PARKING: Max. 2 vehicles per site

FEE: $16/night

RESTRICTIONS: *Pets:* Must be leashed
Quiet Hours: 10 p.m.– 6 a.m.
Visitors: Max. 6 people per site
Fires: In provided grills
Alcohol: Prohibited
Stay Limit: 14 days per year, limited to 7 days Memorial Day–Labor Day
Other: Max. 3 tents per site; check-out time is noon

MAP

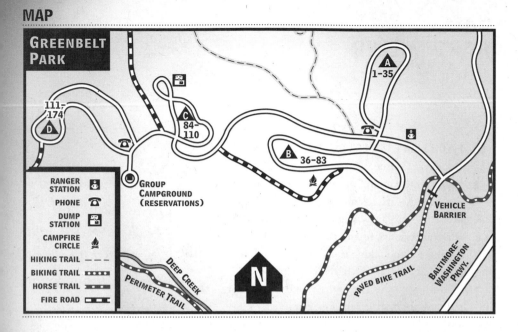

GREENBELT PARK

A 1-35

D 111-174

C 84-110

B 36-83

| RANGER STATION |
| PHONE |
| DUMP STATION |
| CAMPFIRE CIRCLE |
| HIKING TRAIL |
| BIKING TRAIL |
| HORSE TRAIL |
| FIRE ROAD |

GROUP CAMPGROUND (RESERVATIONS)

VEHICLE BARRIER

DEEP CREEK

PERIMETER TRAIL

PAVED BIKE TRAIL

BALTIMORE-WASHINGTON PKWY.

N

GETTING THERE

From I-95, take Exit 23 (MD Route 201, Kenilworth Avenue South) to Greenbelt Road East (MD Route 193). The park is a quarter-mile down on the right.

GPS COORDINATES

UTM Zone (NAD27) 18S
Easting 334987
Northing 4316177

34
HART-MILLER
ISLAND

IF YOU WANT TO FEEL like a modern day Robinson Crusoe, take a boat to Hart-Miller Island, at the mouth of the Back River in the Chesapeake Bay. OK, it's not so remote that you'll feel like that famous castaway, but camping at Hart-Miller is a unique experience in any case.

There are some hiking trails on the island, but they're few, and at 244 acres the park can be exhausted fairly easily. The entire island is considerably larger, more than 1,100 acres, but much of it is off-limits. So don't expect oodles of recreation. Still, this isn't why people go to the island. If you've spent the day kayaking the area and want a place to stop, fish, swim, and then pitch your tent under the stars and listen to the soft lap of small waves, you couldn't pick a better location.

The U.S. Army Corps of Engineers began constructing Hart-Miller in 1981 using dredged materials from Baltimore Harbor and the channels leading to and from. Large wildlife restoration projects, some still ongoing, account for the disparity in size between the park and the larger island. Projects include recreating forest, ponds, and habitat for migratory shorebirds, including wetlands and mudflats. Although the projects won't be completed entirely until 2009 at the earliest, Hart-Miller is already a place of major importance for migrating birds. Some 20,000 waterfowl have at times been seen on the island. Sandpipers and plovers share space with Caspian Terns.

Don't be turned off by the fact that you must take a private boat to camp here. Getting to Hart-Miller is easy. The smallest of vessels—kayak or canoe is perfect—will get you there without a problem. From Rocky Point Marina, the logical debarkation for Hart-Miller, it's less than 1.5 miles of easy paddling. This does, however, account for the low security rating above.

> *If you want a place to fish, swim, and then pitch your tent under the stars and listen to the soft lap of small waves, you couldn't pick a better location.*

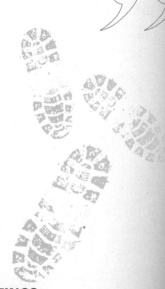

RATINGS

Beauty: ✪ ✪ ✪ ✪ ✪
Privacy: ✪ ✪ ✪ ✪ ✪
Spaciousness: ✪ ✪ ✪ ✪ ✪
Quiet: ✪ ✪ ✪ ✪ ✪
Security: ✪ ✪
Cleanliness: ✪ ✪ ✪ ✪

KEY INFORMATION

ADDRESS: Hart-Miller Island
State Park
c/o Gunpowder Falls
State Park
2813 Jerusalem Road
P.O. Box 480
Kingsville, MD 21087
(410) 592-2897

OPERATED BY: Maryland Department of Natural
Resources

OPEN: Last weekend in
March–Labor Day

SITES: Indeterminate—pitch
your tent where
there's space

EACH SITE HAS: Primitive; there are
picnic tables and fire
rings on the island

ASSIGNMENT: First come, first
served

REGISTRATION: Rangers will collect
fee when they visit
the island

FACILITIES: Portable toilet,
picnic tables

PARKING: None

FEE: $6/night

RESTRICTIONS: *Pets:* None
Quiet Hours: None
official, but rangers
ask for courtesy
toward all visitors
Visitors: No policy
Fires: In fire rings
Alcohol: Not
permitted
Stay Limit: None
Other: Access only by
private boat

I've never heard of any major problems at Hart-Miller, and neither had the ranger I spoke to, but the possibility exists of someone boating to the island and causing trouble. With no easy access back to land, the consequences could be serious. That said, don't let such a remote possibility dissuade you from camping at this unique spot.

To get to Hart-Miller, park to the right just after the Rocky Point entrance (gates are open even after the park closes and you can leave your car there overnight). The ramp is at the end of the parking lot. Once in the water, swing around to the left; you'll pass North Point and then Pleasure Island. Hart-Miller is next. You'll see a mooring area as you approach to the right. A beautiful beach tempts, and the primitive sites will soon come into view. Some are crudely marked, but the standing rule is that you can pitch your tent wherever there is space—and you can probably count on there being space.

MAP

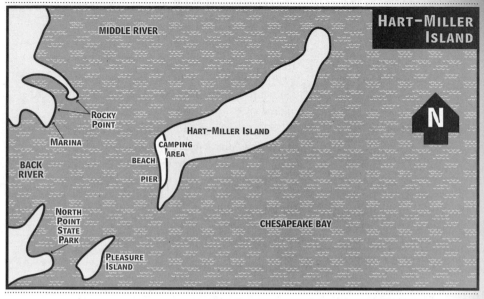

MIDDLE RIVER

HART–MILLER
ISLAND

ROCKY
POINT

MARINA

HART–MILLER ISLAND

CAMPING
AREA

BACK
RIVER

BEACH

PIER

NORTH
POINT
STATE
PARK

CHESAPEAKE BAY

PLEASURE
ISLAND

N

GETTING THERE

To Rocky Point Marina:
Take I-695 to Exit 35,
Southeast Boulevard (MD
Route 702) south. Follow
Route 702 until it merges
right, into Back River Neck
Road. Take a left onto
Barrison Point Road and a
right onto Rocky Point Road.

GPS COORDINATES

UTM Zone (NAD27) 18S
Easting 381834
Northing 4345917

35
LITTLE BENNETT REGIONAL PARK

LITTLE BENNETT REGIONAL PARK has developed a loyal following among D.C.-area families looking for a quick and easy escape. Even the most extreme adventurer has to appreciate the 20-plus miles of trails within this 3,600-acre park that can be reached from either Baltimore or Washington in less than an hour.

The Hawk's Reach Activity Center serves as the park's center of activities, coordinating nature hikes, children's crafts, socials, and other family-geared entertainment. It also houses a popular game room. Large playgrounds, soccer fields, horseshoe pits, and volleyball courts provide additional entertainment and recreation for campers. I realize that the description above makes Little Bennett sound like a day camp swarming with kids and burned-out adults. It's really much more pleasant than that; there's a sincere appreciation for the place that ripples through its users. In a county that is increasingly suburbanized, this little slice of the natural world is cherished. Several folks I spoke to described it as the perfect family camping spot—easy to get to and easy to love once you're there. The friendly staff assures it remains safe and full of activities. It's also extremely well maintained, with the sparkling-clean bathhouses being just one indication of that.

With so much wooded land within, Little Bennett manages to be quiet and serene, even with all the activity and recreation. In fact, hiking some of the outer trails can easily leave you feeling like the woods are yours alone. Additionally, the campsites are well wooded and nicely spaced.

Little Bennett's campsites are logically arranged, offering slightly different experiences for each loop depending on size and want. Loop A comes first, with sites 1 to 20. Loop B, slightly smaller, contains sites 21 to 34. Loop C is the most intimate of all, as it contains

RATINGS

Beauty: ✪ ✪ ✪ ✪
Privacy: ✪ ✪ ✪
Spaciousness: ✪ ✪ ✪ ✪ ✪
Quiet: ✪ ✪ ✪ ✪
Security: ✪ ✪ ✪ ✪ ✪
Cleanliness: ✪ ✪ ✪ ✪ ✪

only 13 sites (35 to 47). Loop D, the park's electric loop, sits right across the road and contains sites 48 to 72. Loop E, my favorite, contains sites 73 to 91. If you do stay in Loop E, try for Site 85; it sits next to the Bennett Ridge Trail, which you can take to access the Beaver Valley Trail toward a beautiful spot at Little Bennett Creek. (There's an excellent trail map available at the Contact Station). Sites 83 and 81 are also nice. If you have little kids with you, try for the internal sites on E: 74, 76, 78, 80, 82, 84, 86, 89, and 91. All these give easy access to the playground in the loop without crossing the camp road.

Other particularly nice sites include 13, 15, 17, 19, and 20 in Loop A and 41, 43, and 45 in Loop C.

KEY INFORMATION

ADDRESS:	Little Bennett Regional Park Campground
	23701 Frederick Road
	Clarksburg, MD 20871
	(301) 972-6581
OPERATED BY:	Maryland National Capital Park and Planning Commission
OPEN:	April 1–October 31; also open for weekend camping in March and November
EACH SITE HAS:	Parking pad, picnic table, fire ring; many sites have a tent pad and a lantern post
ASSIGNMENT:	Reservations recommended, accepted after January 1 for any dates during that year's camping season
REGISTRATION:	Call (301) 972-9222 or register on site at the Contact Station
FACILITIES:	Dump station, comfort stations, laundry room, activity and nature center, playgrounds, ball fields, camp store
PARKING:	Max. 2 vehicles per site
FEE:	$21/night, $29 electric
RESTRICTIONS:	*Pets:* Permitted on leash
	Quiet Hours: 11 p.m.–6 a.m.
	Visitors: Max. 6 people per site; visitors must register and pay at the Contact Station
	Fires: In fire ring
	Alcohol: Not allowed
	Stay Limit: 2 weeks
	Other: Check-in after 1 p.m., check-out 11 a.m.

MAP

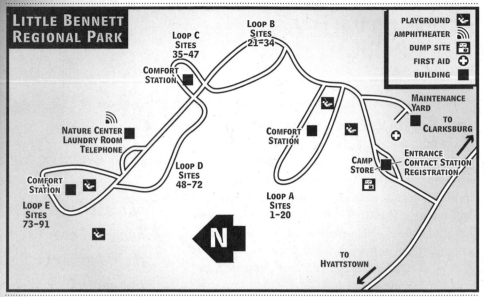

GETTING THERE

Take I-270 to Exit 18, MD Route 121, Clarksburg Road North. Take a left on MD Route 355, Frederick Road.

GPS COORDINATES

UTM Zone (NAD27) 18S
Easting 302388
Northing 4346781

36
PATAPSCO VALLEY STATE PARK:
HILTON AREA

PATAPSCO VALLEY STATE PARK (PVSP), straddling the Patapsco River and encompassing
sections of four counties, can rightly be considered central Maryland's recreation granddaddy.
Sprawling over 32 miles of the Patapsco River and
encompassing 14,000 acres, PVSP possesses numerous
hiking trails and an abundance of outdoor recreation
activities within its five developed areas. Aside from its
great reputation for hiking, PVSP offers fantastic fishing and mountain biking. Its location amidst heavy
population centers makes it a true haven for nature-
seekers (many sections are entirely devoid of people
and feel very remote and wild). Those who haven't
been to the park might never guess the beauty and
solitude one can easily find simply by walking a mile
or two (or less). It's a haven for families who want a
couple of nights away from home but want to reach
their destination in a few minutes. For these folks, even
the occasional rumble of a train traversing the parkland is a small price to pay for the abundance of activities available and the ability to sleep safely in nature
just a few miles from home.

I know PVSP from hiking its many trails (more
than 170 miles in all), and I used to be rather snobbish
about regarding it as a camping destination: too busy,
too crowded, etc. However, I must admit to being very
pleasantly surprised the first time I visited the Hilton
Area's campground. It's a gem, far from the main
action centers elsewhere in the park. It's also small and
very well wooded, assuring quiet and privacy that can
be tough to get otherwise.

Hilton's chief attraction is its diminutive size and
its nonelectric status. Additionally, it sits near some
great hiking trails. One of my favorites remains the
yellow-blazed Buzzards Rock Trail. This stunning trail
can be reached very easily from the campground,

> *It's a haven for fami-
> lies who want a couple
> of nights away from
> home but want to reach
> their destination in a
> few minutes.*

RATINGS

Beauty: ✪ ✪ ✪ ✪
Privacy: ✪ ✪ ✪ ✪
Spaciousness: ✪ ✪ ✪
Quiet: ✪ ✪ ✪ ✪
Security: ✪ ✪ ✪ ✪ ✪
Cleanliness: ✪ ✪ ✪ ✪ ✪

KEY INFORMATION

ADDRESS: Patapsco Valley
State Park
8020 Baltimore
National Pike
Ellicott City, MD
21043
(410) 461-5005

OPERATED BY: Maryland Department of Natural
Resources

OPEN: April–September

SITES: 12, plus 6 mini-cabins
and 1 camp host

EACH SITE HAS: Picnic table, fire
ring, lantern post

ASSIGNMENT: Self-registration for
walk-ins, but
advanced reservations recommended

REGISTRATION: (888) 432-CAMP
(2267), or online at
http://reservations
/dnr.state.md.us

FACILITIES: Playground, bathhouse, picnic area

PARKING: Only on camp pad,
2 vehicles max.

FEE: $20/night, $25/night
electric

RESTRICTIONS: *Pets:* Not allowed
Quiet Hours: 11 p.m.–
7 a.m.
Visitors: Must register
and must leave by
9:30 p.m.; max. 6
people per site
Fires: In fire rings
Alcohol: Allowed
Stay Limit: 2-week
maximum; 2-night
minimum Memorial
Day–Labor Day
Other: No self-
registration before
1 p.m. or on Friday
and Saturday; can
self-register for only
1 night at a time;
camping groups must
have at least one 18
years old; Check-out
1 p.m.

which is surrounded by woods and more trails on all sides: Charcoal to the west, Santee Branch to the south and east, and Sawmill Branch to the north. The Sawmill Branch Trail ends at the Buzzards Rock Trail, just before the stone CSX bridge and the paved Grist Mill Trail.

Buzzards Rock heads precipitously uphill and leads to (and then passes) the rock for which the trail is named. Buzzards used to congregate here because the site commands a view of the valley—and the prey lurking in the woods. It's spectacular, especially in the fall. Because it requires a hefty climb, I often have it to myself when I'm here. If you've brought your bike, the paved Grist Mill Trail follows the Patapsco River and eventually passes Lost Lake, a fishing lake reserved for those over 61 or under 16 years of age or with disabilities.

Oddly, I find the Hilton campground often quite empty. I think locals see the Hilton area of PVSP mostly as a day-use area. Hilton has 12 tent-only campsites, plus one reserved for the camp host. Campers requiring heat and electricity can rent one of the six camper cabins. To avoid the light coming from the cabins, choose sites farthest away; sites 277 and 278 are closest. Be aware that there's a power line cut behind sites 276 and 277, so they are a bit more open than the others. But even these are pleasant sites. Thick, mature trees surround all 12, and all sit on the outside of the camp loop, while the bathhouse is on the inside. In short, my snobbishness was totally unwarranted—this is a very pleasant campground.

MAP

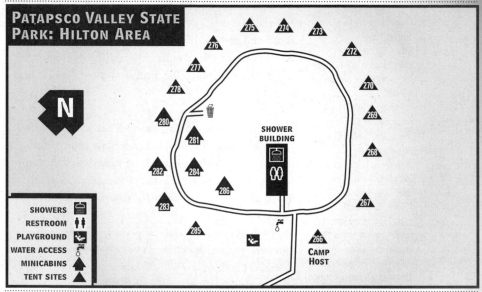

PATAPSCO VALLEY STATE PARK: HILTON AREA

275 274 273
276 272
277
278 270
280 269
281
SHOWER BUILDING
268
282 284
286
267
283
285
266
CAMP HOST

SHOWERS
RESTROOM
PLAYGROUND
WATER ACCESS
MINICABINS
TENT SITES

Take I-695 to Exit 13, Frederick Road, toward Catonsville to a left on South Rolling Road. Go straight at the big leftward curve onto Hilton Avenue. Park is 1.5 miles on the right.

GPS COORDINATES

UTM Zone (NAD27) 18S
Easting 349013
Northing 4346017

> *In short, a place where kids (and their parents) can keep themselves happily entertained for days.*

DESPITE ITS CROWDED FEEL (or maybe because of it), Patapsco Valley State Park (PVSP) is a logical camping destination for families, especially those with little kids. I have two very young daughters, who aren't quite ready for camping yet, but PVSP will be my first destination when they are. The reason is simple: if it doesn't work out, we can easily pack up and make the short trip home. Another attraction for people in a similar situation is that they can hop into the car and pick up any forgotten supplies in nearby towns.

When you enter the park's Hollofield area, you'll reach what many consider to be PVSP's epicenter. Within a short radius, you'll find a popular vista, playgrounds and picnic areas, hiking trails, and the park headquarters. The number of day-users here can get thick, and you have to walk north to reach uncrowded trails. But once there, the Ole Ranger and Peaceful Pond trails are fantastic, marked by sloping, wooded hills rising above the Patapsco River gorge. To enjoy all the features that make PVSP so attractive, you might find that you'll have to head south toward the Hilton, Avalon, Orange Grove, and Glen Artney areas. Once that easy trip is complete (and you can do it by floating down the river), there's a ton to do: boating, fishing, hiking, hunting, horseback riding, mountain biking, and nature and history programs put on by park rangers. In short, a place where kids (and their parents) can keep themselves happily entertained for days.

From the popular overlook, the campground is to the right, down the hill and past the pavilions and boathouses. On the way to the campground, you'll pass the fabulous River Ridge Trail. One drawback to this day-use section is that it sits very close to Route 40 and road noise is pretty bad. But the campground is fairly far from the road; all you should hear is the

RATINGS

Beauty: ✪ ✪ ✪ ✪
Privacy: ✪ ✪ ✪
Spaciousness: ✪ ✪ ✪
Quiet: ✪ ✪ ✪
Security: ✪ ✪ ✪ ✪ ✪
Cleanliness: ✪ ✪ ✪ ✪

occasional truck or motorcycle.

Of PVSP's two campgrounds, Hollofield is the busier. It has 73 sites (400 to 472), including a pet loop. The pet loop includes sites 461 to 472. Pets are also allowed at sites 400 to 403. If you have a pet, go for Site 465, which is very private. If you don't have a pet, no worries: the pet loop is far from other sites, so you shouldn't be disturbed. Though this might seem counterintuitive, it might not be a bad idea to head straight to the pet loop even if you don't have a pet; it's smaller and more private than the main campground section. If doggies are controlled, your chances for quiet might actually increase in the pet loop.

All other sites sit north, on one big loop. In this loop, sites 405, 406, and 425 are wheelchair accessible. Nonelectric sites are 430 to 472; of these, 430 to 460 are tent-only. Electric sites include 400 to 403 and 405 to 429, with 404 reserved for the camp host. After the tent-only area, sites 461 to 472 sit off by themselves in an area that hosts a multitude of deer. Sites 434 to 449 sit on the farthest edges of the loop, so they won't see much through traffic and are a little more private. Of these, I like 448, which sits by itself.

KEY INFORMATION

ADDRESS:	Patapsco Valley State Park
	8020 Baltimore National Pike
	Ellicott City, MD 21043
	(410) 461-5005
OPERATED BY:	Maryland Department of Natural Resources
OPEN:	Last weekend in April–October
SITES:	73
EACH SITE HAS:	Camp pad, picnic table, fire ring
ASSIGNMENT:	Advanced reservations recommended, but same-day self-registration is allowed
REGISTRATION:	If self-registering, go to camp headquarters, open 9 a.m.–3 p.m. Monday–Friday; if no one is there, self-register by choosing available site and registering at the info desk. For advance reservations, call (888) 432-CAMP (2267) or go to http://reservations.dnr.state.md.us.
FACILITIES:	Bathhouses, camp store, playground, visitor center, frost-free spigot
PARKING:	Only on camp pad, 2 vehicles max.
FEE:	$20/night, $25/night electric
RESTRICTIONS:	*Pets:* On sites 400–403 and 461–472; must be leashed
	Quiet Hours: 11 p.m.–7 a.m.
	Visitors: Visitors must register and leave by 9:30 p.m.; max. 6 people per site
	Fires: In fire rings
	Alcohol: Allowed
	Stay Limit: Max. 2 weeks
	Other: No self-registration before 1 p.m. or on Friday and Saturday; can self-register for only 1 night at a time; camping groups must have at least one 18 years old; check-out is 1 p.m.

MAP

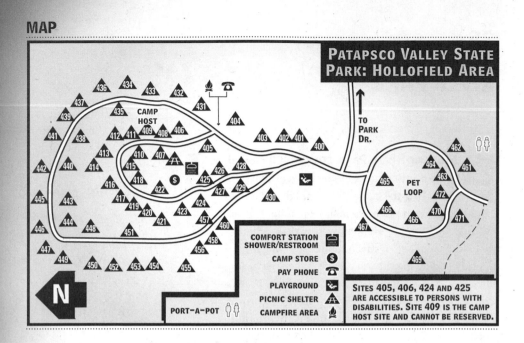

PATAPSCO VALLEY STATE PARK: HOLLOFIELD AREA

CAMP HOST

TO PARK DR.

PET LOOP

COMFORT STATION SHOWER/RESTROOM	
CAMP STORE	$
PAY PHONE	☎
PLAYGROUND	
PICNIC SHELTER	⛺
CAMPFIRE AREA	

PORT-A-POT

N

SITES 405, 406, 424 AND 425 ARE ACCESSIBLE TO PERSONS WITH DISABILITIES. SITE 409 IS THE CAMP HOST SITE AND CANNOT BE RESERVED.

GETTING THERE

Take I-695 to Exit 14, MD Route 40 West. Once over the Patapsco River Bridge, turn right.

GPS COORDINATES

UTM Zone (NAD27) 18S
Easting 345709
Northing 4350152

PATUXENT RIVER PARK COMPRISES more than 6,000 acres of environmentally sensitive parkland along the eastern edge of Prince George's County. I grew up not more than half an hour from this park and I didn't even know it existed. When I sheepishly admitted as much to the park ranger (quickly adding that I hadn't lived in the area in some fifteen years), he laughed off my "confession." "We're Prince George's County's best-kept secret," he said. Apparently, even many residents in nearby Marlton don't know of it either. Part of the reason for this is intentional: the park operates under a "limited-use" policy, meaning that users must register and receive permits for all activities.

> *To say your space will be large is the understatement of the century.*

I'm a bit hesitant to give up the secret, now that I've been there. It is an absolute jewel. Aside from the stunning natural area, the camping setup is a dream. There are six campsites total, but that number is misleading. Each site can accommodate dozens of campers; the park has hosted a couple of hundred campers before. (It's probably wise to ask if there are groups scheduled to camp in the airfield. If so, ask for a spot far away.) But if you reserve a spot—even if you are camping alone—you get the site all to yourself. To say your space will be large is the understatement of the century. Five campsites are spread out along the edge of the defunct Croom Airfield, a large open field, and the distance between them is immense. For so much space and so much natural beauty, the price should be exorbitant. Instead, it's a few bucks, plus a ten-dollar refundable deposit. That money gets you a key to open the gate for the camping area as well as an on-site trailer. The trailer has bathrooms inside, which are kept nice and clean. There's also a game room, with basketballs, volleyballs, soccer balls, and horseshoes. There are eight miles of trails for hikers and equestrian use, as well as on-site

RATINGS

Beauty: ✩ ✩ ✩ ✩
Privacy: ✩ ✩ ✩ ✩ ✩
Spaciousness: ✩ ✩ ✩ ✩ ✩
Quiet: ✩ ✩ ✩ ✩
Security: ✩ ✩ ✩ ✩ ✩
Cleanliness: ✩ ✩ ✩ ✩ ✩

ADDRESS: Patuxent River Park
16000 Croom
Airport Road
Upper Marlboro,
MD 20772
(301) 627-6074

OPERATED BY: Maryland-National
Capital Park
and Planning
Commission

OPEN: Airfield is year-
round; canoe site
April–October

SITES: 6

EACH SITE HAS: Fire pit and picnic
tables

ASSIGNMENT: Reservations
required

REGISTRATION: Call the park at
(301) 627-6074
Tuesday–Friday, 8:30
a.m.–4 p.m.

FACILITIES: Flush toilets, wildlife
center, boat launch
and rental, museums

PARKING: At the barn in the
airfield, on site for
canoe site

FEE: $3 Prince George's
and Montgomery
County residents;
$4 all others. Boat
rental: $17 residents,
$20 others

RESTRICTIONS: *Pets:* Allowed
Quiet Hours: None
Visitors: Airfield sites
can accommodate
up to 200, canoe site
up to 20
Fires: In fire rings
only
Alcohol: Prohibited
Stay Limit: None
Other: Water must be
obtained in the
group camping site.

museums. Additionally, the park supplies water and firewood. There's a potential drawback in that if you're camping alongside two hundred Scouts, it might be unpleasant. However, the chances are just as good that you'll have a huge portion of an airfield to yourself. In either case, it's a bonus that no RVs or trailers are allowed.

As indicated above, there are five campsites in the airfield. Of these, D sits in a wooded copse. A and B are located along the edge of the woods on a little rise above the airfield. C and E are also in the open, but are bordered by woods on either side, so depending on the time of day, these can be shaded as well. Only D is truly shaded, so if that's a priority, be sure to ask for it. I think it's great to be able to walk a little distance into the field and stargaze at night.

The sixth site sits all by itself adjacent to Jug Bay. The Jug Bay Natural Area is designated by the Audubon Society as an "Important Birding Area." More than two-hundred-fifty bird species have been spotted at Jug Bay, and more than one-hundred of these nest in the area. The campsite can accommodate up to twenty campers, and it is truly spectacular. But, like the airfield sites, it takes only one person to reserve the spot. Imagine a wooded campsite with your own personal road (a locked gate on the entrance road and you holding the key), and Jug Bay just 50 yards away from your spot. It's a camper's dream. Admittedly, the site is tough to get on weekends, but the campsite generally remains free during the week. Also, if you can reserve a few months in advance, your chances of getting it for a weekend are decent.

Obviously, most campers at Patuxent River Park wind up in the group camping area, but if you can get the canoe spot, don't hesitate. After paying your nominal fee for the campsite and leaving a $10 refundable deposit for the key, you can drive to the site and lock up behind you. Just beyond the gate, there's a big open parking area, flanking two toilets to the left. A buffer of foliage is next. And Jug Bay sits just beyond that. A little pier juts into the water, where you can launch and fish. Trails wind along the river's edge. Up a small rise to the right, within a thick stand of trees, is the camp

MAP

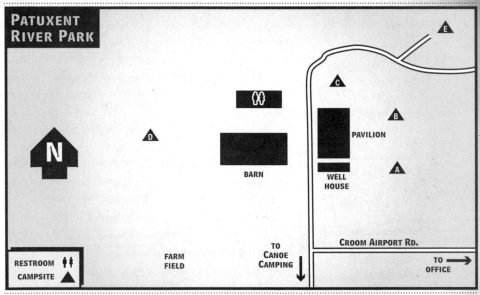

area. Picnic tables and a grill are scattered among several level tent spaces. The camping area is very close to the water, but far enough away so that the large concentrations of biting insects that congregate around the water seem to generally stay away from the tent area ("stay away" being a relative term, of course). You can bring your own canoe, or rent one here. The park even offers guided trips.

GETTING THERE

From Upper Marlboro, take MD Route 301 to Croom Station Road (left turn). Croom Station Road leads to Croom Road. Go left on Croom Road, and turn left onto Croom Airport Road.

GPS COORDINATES

UTM Zone (NAD27) 18S
Easting 351501
Northing 4290561

> *John Smith's 1608 assessment of the area is applicable even today: 'Heaven and earth seemed never to have agreed better to frame a place for man's . . . delightful habitation.'*

THE SUSQUEHANNA WAS FIRST explored by John Smith in 1608. Of course, the native Susquehannock Indians had already been hunting and fishing in the area for centuries. Smith's assessment of the area is applicable even today: "Heaven and earth seemed never to have agreed better to frame a place for man's . . . delightful habitation." True enough, if any local outdoor enthusiast needs a reminder why he or she is lucky to live in this area, Susquehanna State Park provides it. Among the Susquehanna River's impressive numbers: 444 miles, a 13 million acre drainage basin pouring 19 million gallons of freshwater into the Chesapeake Bay every minute, the second largest watershed in the eastern United States.

A major draw for Susquehanna State Park is fishing. Striped, smallmouth, and largemouth bass are abundant. Anglers also catch channel catfish, carp, alewife, pike, and perch. What this means is that folks camping are often up and out early, especially in springtime, during the annual herring and shad runs. If that's your primary motivation too, don't worry. The river is large, and a prime spot can easily be claimed. If your motivation for visiting Susquehanna State Park is hiking, be thrilled. The trails, more than 15 miles worth in all, can be surprisingly empty. One of them heads to the Conowingo Dam, a prime spot for birding. There's also much here in the way of historical attractions: the Rock Run Historic Area includes the still-operational Rock Run Grist Mill (1794), as well as the Rock Run Mansion (1804). There's also the Steppingstone Museum, which includes antique farm implements, restored farmhouse, decoy carving, and blacksmith shop.

The campground contains two loops: Acorn and Beechnut. The three walk-in sites on the Acorn Loop

RATINGS

Beauty: ✿ ✿ ✿ ✿ ✿
Privacy: ✿ ✿ ✿
Spaciousness: ✿ ✿ ✿
Quiet: ✿ ✿ ✿
Security: ✿ ✿ ✿ ✿ ✿
Cleanliness: ✿ ✿ ✿ ✿

(18, 20, and 22) are relatively private and well spaced. But among the recommended sites for privacy is site 19 in Acorn, on the inside portion of the loop from the walk-in sites listed above. Generally speaking, the campsites are pretty private and well spaced, so it's tough to find a bad spot in the Acorn Loop. Still, my favorite in Acorn is site 24, which requires a hike-in of about 250 feet. If you can possibly get this site, take it; it's a real beauty.

Sites in the Beechnut Loop are not much different from Acorn. But if you do go there, consider park staff recommendations of sites 5, 10, and 18—these are really nice sites, each guaranteeing a decent amount of privacy. Of these, Site 18 is a walk-in site. The sites best avoided are the ones closest to the electric sites (5 to 10 in Acorn); this means avoid 1 through 3, 11, and 12 in Acorn. Beechnut seems to be the more rugged and remote-feeling of the two loops. The better sites are congregated along the southern edge of the loop.

KEY INFORMATION

ADDRESS: **Susquehanna State Park**
c/o Rocks State Park
3318 Rocks Chrome Hill Road
Jarrettsville, MD 21084
(410) 557-7994 (park headquarters), (410) 734-9035 (campground)

OPERATED BY: **Maryland Department of Natural Resources**

OPEN: **End of April–end of September**

SITES: **69 total (4 walk-in, 6 camper cabins)**

EACH SITE HAS: **Picnic table, fire pit, lantern hook**

ASSIGNMENT: **Sites 18, 20, 22 on the Acorn Loop and Site 29 on the Beechnut Loop are walk-in; reserve all others**

REGISTRATION: **(888) 432-2267 or at http://reservations.dnr.state.md.us**

FACILITIES: **Bathhouse, water, boat launch, playground, picnic areas, pavilions, bow-hunting area, archery range**

PARKING: **On gravel driveway**

FEE: **$20/night, $25/night electric; boat launch, $10/vehicle, $11 out-of-state residents**

RESTRICTIONS: *Pets:* **Must be leashed**
Quiet Hours: **11 p.m.–7 a.m.**
Visitors: **6 people, 2 tents per site (charge of $3 per person over maximum)**
Fires: **In fire rings**
Alcohol: **Permitted at site**
Stay Limit: **2-day minimum Memorial Day–Labor Day on weekends, unless walk-in**
Other: **A Chesapeake Bay Sports Fishing License (tidal license) is required to fish the Susquehanna from Conowingo Dam to the Chesapeake**

MAP

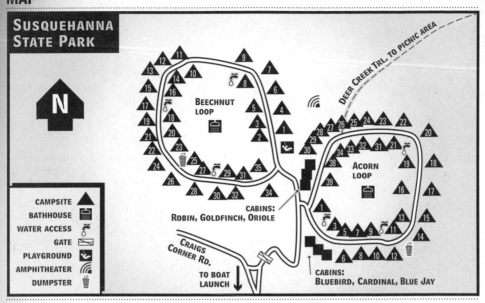

SUSQUEHANNA STATE PARK

N

BEECHNUT LOOP

ACORN LOOP

DEER CREEK TRL. TO PICNIC AREA

CABINS: ROBIN, GOLDFINCH, ORIOLE

CRAIGS CORNER RD.

TO BOAT LAUNCH

CABINS: BLUEBIRD, CARDINAL, BLUE JAY

CAMPSITE	
BATHHOUSE	
WATER ACCESS	
GATE	
PLAYGROUND	
AMPHITHEATER	
DUMPSTER	

GETTING THERE

Take I-95 to Exit 89, MD Route 155 West. Go 2.5 miles to a right on MD Route 161. Go 0.3 miles to a right on Rock Run Road and follow Rock Run into the park. Follow signs to camping area.

GPS COORDINATES

UTM Zone (NAD27) 18S
Easting 399468
Northing 4385328

SOUTHERN MARYLAND AND EASTERN SHORE

40
ASSATEAGUE ISLAND NATIONAL SEASHORE:
BAYSIDE CAMPGROUND

ASSATEAGUE ISLAND IS A BARRIER ISLAND, stretching 37 miles from just south of Ocean City all the way to Chincoteague in Virginia. It's very narrow in places; this allows for watching the sunrise over the Atlantic and then turning around later in the day and watching it set over Sinepuxent or Chincoteague Bay.

The name Assateague is known all over the country as the "place with the wild horses." Indeed—they're all over the island, though the Virginia (known as Chincoteague ponies) and Maryland herds are kept separated. First-time visitors to Assateague are often amazed when they spot one of the animals; by the end of the visit, they've probably fought more than one urge to shoo them away from their campsite or off the road. The horses have certainly gotten used to humans and show no fear (I still have a vivid memory of being horrified when, as a little boy, I was in the back seat of a car when one stuck his snout in the window and held it inches from my face). The horses are stout (read: short and fat) and don't inspire images of free-riding Western plains Wildfires. Still, they are a sight. Their presence makes Assateague a truly special place, and certainly a must-camp destination for any Marylander. Though natives make up the bulk of Assateague's campers, you'll find visitors from all over the country.

Assateague Island National Seashore is divided into two separate camping areas: Oceanside and Bayside, logically named because of their respective locations. The Oceanside has double the sites because it's more popular. Nevertheless, campers—especially repeat campers who always go for the oceanside sites—should give the bayside a try. Certainly, if you desire shade in the hot summer months, the bayside sites provide much more of it than the oceanside ones, which offer virtually none. However, it is much more buggy in the

> *The name Assateague is known all over the country as the 'place with the wild horses.'*

RATINGS

Beauty: ✿ ✿ ✿ ✿ ✿
Privacy: ✿ ✿ ✿
Spaciousness: ✿ ✿ ✿
Quiet: ✿ ✿ ✿
Security: ✿ ✿ ✿ ✿ ✿
Cleanliness: ✿ ✿ ✿ ✿

summer on the bayside. This detriment, combined with the magnetic pull of the ocean, means that the bayside is often the consolation for those who couldn't get an oceanside site. However, there are some real advantages to the bayside sites. If your reasons for coming include wildlife-viewing, birding, or canoeing/kayaking, the bayside is the much better bet. Because of the increased vegetation, the area is a birder's paradise. Plus, the bayside has the national seashore's boat launch and you can have fires in the fire pits on the bayside (there are only grills at the oceanside campsites).

The Bayside Campground has three loops: A, B, and C. Each of the three loops has a shower and restroom. A very nice feature of the Bayside Campground is the bicycle and canoe rental, at the westernmost end of the campground, past Loop C at the Bayside Picnic Area. Loop A has sites 1 to 24, B has 25 to 37, and C contains 38 to 49, so no lone loop is terribly big. Generators are prohibited in Loop B; if you want some quiet, shoot for Loop B. The best site in the campground is in B: Site 35. It overlooks a beautiful little sandy beach. If you can't get 35, try to get one of nearby ones (33 to 37).

Since the Sinepuxent Bay wraps around the entire peninsula where the bayside sites are located, no one site is very far from the water. However, the main camp road does sit between some sites and the bay. If you want a site without that barrier, go for the sites on the western side of the three loops. Specifically, this means 14, 15, 17, 18, 20, 22, and 24

KEY INFORMATION

ADDRESS:	Assateague Island National Seashore
	7206 National Seashore Lane
	Berlin, MD 21811
	(410) 641-3030
OPERATED BY:	National Park Service
OPEN:	All year. Note: Bayside Campground closed for renovations until June 1, 2008
SITES:	49
EACH SITE HAS:	Picnic table, grill, fire ring
ASSIGNMENT:	First come, first served mid-October–mid-April, reservations recommended the rest of year
REGISTRATION:	Register at the North Beach Ranger Station, or call (800) 365-CAMP, or online at http://reservations.nps.gov
FACILITIES:	Chemical toilets, cold-water showers, drinking water
PARKING:	2 vehicles total; parking areas off Bayberry Drive for walk-in sites
FEE:	Mid-October–mid-April, $16/night, rest of year, $20/night
RESTRICTIONS:	*Pets:* Permitted, but must be attended
	Quiet Hours: 10 p.m.–6 a.m.
	Visitors: 6 persons (or immediate family) max.
	Fires: In fire rings
	Alcohol: Not permitted
	Stay Limit: Total of 30 nights per year, only 14 during reservation season
	Other: Illegal to feed or approach wildlife ($500 fine); check-in and check-out at noon

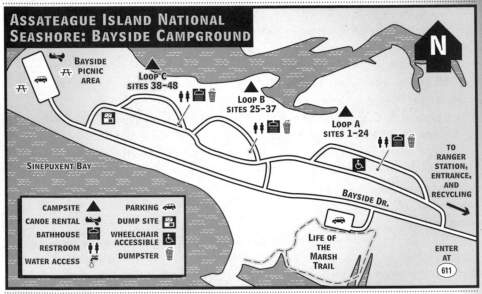

in Loop A (of these, sites 22 and 24 are closest); 33, 35, and 37 in Loop B; and 45, 46, and 48 in Loop C (though 47 and 49 aren't bad either).

Take US Route 50 just before Ocean City to MD 611 South.

UTM Zone (NAD27) 18S

Easting 486454

Northing 4228746

> *How'd you like to wake up on the beach, the Atlantic Ocean over the closest dune, while the silhouette of a wild horse stretches across your tent wall?*

HOW'D YOU LIKE TO WAKE UP on the beach, the Atlantic Ocean over the closest dune, while the silhouette of a wild horse stretches across your tent wall? Sounds like paradise? It's pretty close, and it's well worth the relentless mosquitoes. It's Assateague Island National Seashore.

Oceanside campsites at Assateague Island can be tough to get. Everyone's clamoring for a spot in the sand just a hundred feet from the Atlantic. (You should note, however, that the campsites are in the dunes, so the ocean won't be visible from your tent.) Even summer's heat and biting bugs aren't enough to deter the crowds. They come for the sunrises, sunsets, horses, swimming, fishing, crabbing, boating, and off-roading.

Though not as much of a draw, hiking is a must, but for those not used to walking along a barrier island, there are some must-know things. One of my earliest memories involves hiking out in nearby Toms Cove (on Chincoteague Island, in Virginia) during a trip to Assateague; we walked and walked, seemingly for miles, and the water barely reached up to our waists. Then, quite suddenly, it got higher and higher as we ran back, barely reaching shore before the water was over our heads. Also, so much standing water brings out mosquitoes in droves. Gnats and ticks are constant pests as well. Wind is something else people complain about. Make sure to bring sand stakes for your tent—short stakes could very well mean your tent gets blown away.

Nevertheless, the crowds come, and if you've camped here, it's easy to see why. Without question, the best bets are the oceanside walk-in sites. These are tent-only and are all within 200 feet of parking areas. It's a great setup. Leave your car at the lot, and then walk to the site, right on the beach. Some privacy is lost, but this is a natural function of the topography—in

RATINGS

Beauty: ✿ ✿ ✿ ✿ ✿
Privacy: ✿ ✿ ✿
Spaciousness: ✿ ✿ ✿
Quiet: ✿ ✿ ✿
Security: ✿ ✿ ✿ ✿ ✿
Cleanliness: ✿ ✿ ✿ ✿

most cases, sand separates you and the next tent, as opposed to a tree buffer. However, the sites are surprisingly well spaced and can even feel private. The oceanside walk-ins number 42 to 104. The best of the best are sites 99 to 104 (more private), which lie on the eastern end of the Oceanside Area, on South Ocean Beach, and leave virtually nothing between you and the ocean. The Life of the Dunes Nature Trail sits at the end of this area, beyond the camp roads.

Also included in the Oceanside Campground are Loop 1 (sites 1 to 19) and Loop 2 (sites 20 to 41); these loops are drive-in. The pleasant Life of the Forest Trail sits across Oceanside Campground Drive and Bayberry Drive from sites 20 to 24 in the drive-in section and 42 to 46 of the walk-in area. (There's also a Life of the Marsh nature trail, off Bayside Drive, near the Bayside camping area.) There are six well-spaced shower-and-restroom facilities strewn about the Oceanside Campground. Additionally, a wheelchair-accessible trail to the beach can be found between sites 7 and 9 in Loop 1.

Again, getting a site in the popular months is tough enough (book as far in advance as you can), so take what's available. But if you do have your pick of spots, the proximity to certain activities might be what leads you in a certain direction. For instance, while you can dive into the Atlantic anywhere you like, a lifeguard beach (North Ocean Beach) sits closest to the entrance to Loop One; if you've got little kids, this might be the wisest choice. If you want more privacy and easy access to the trails along the island heading

KEY INFORMATION

ADDRESS:	Assateague Island National Seashore
	7206 National Seashore Lane
	Berlin, MD 21811
	(410) 641-3030
OPERATED BY:	National Park Service
OPEN:	All year
SITES:	104
EACH SITE HAS:	Picnic table, upright grill
ASSIGNMENT:	First come, first served mid-October–mid-April, reservations recommended the rest of year
REGISTRATION:	Self-register at the North Beach Ranger Station, or call (800) 365-CAMP, or register online at http://reservations.nps.gov
FACILITIES:	Chemical toilets, cold-water showers, drinking water
PARKING:	2 vehicles total; parking areas off Bayberry Drive for walk-in sites
FEE:	Mid-October–mid-April, $16/night; rest of the year, $20/night
RESTRICTIONS:	*Pets:* Permitted, but must be attended
	Quiet Hours: 10 p.m.–6 a.m.
	Visitors: 6 persons (or immediate family) max.
	Fires: Allowed on beach below the high-tide line but not at sites
	Alcohol: Not permitted
	Stay Limit: Total of 30 nights per year, only 14 during reservation season
	Other: Illegal to feed or approach wildlife ($500 fine); check-in and check-out at noon

MAP

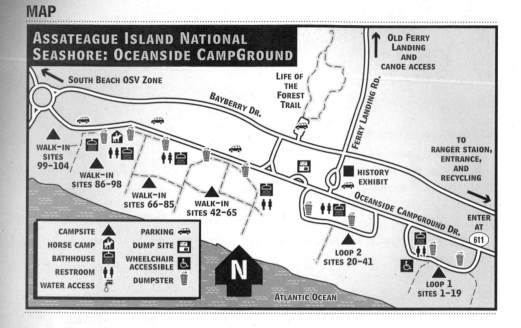

ASSATEAGUE ISLAND NATIONAL SEASHORE: OCEANSIDE CAMPGROUND

SOUTH BEACH OSV ZONE

OLD FERRY LANDING AND CANOE ACCESS

BAYBERRY DR.

LIFE OF THE FOREST TRAIL

FERRY LANDING RD.

WALK-IN SITES 99-104

WALK-IN SITES 86-98

WALK-IN SITES 66-85

WALK-IN SITES 42-65

HISTORY EXHIBIT

TO RANGER STAION, ENTRANCE, AND RECYCLING

OCEANSIDE CAMPGROUND DR.

ENTER AT 611

LOOP 2 SITES 20-41

LOOP 1 SITES 1-19

CAMPSITE	PARKING
HORSE CAMP	DUMP SITE
BATHHOUSE	WHEELCHAIR ACCESSIBLE
RESTROOM	DUMPSTER
WATER ACCESS	

N

ATLANTIC OCEAN

GETTING THERE

Take US Route 50 just before Ocean City to MD 611 South.

south toward Chincoteague, go for the tent-only sites at the end of the loop, on South Ocean Beach. Last, if clamming, crabbing, and boating are more your thing, the road to Old Ferry Landing sits across from Loop 2, past the visitor center (well worth a visit itself).

GPS COORDINATES

UTM Zone (NAD27) 18S
Easting 486643
Northing 4228488

42
ASSATEAGUE ISLAND NATIONAL SEASHORE:
BACKCOUNTRY SITES

THE BACKCOUNTRY CAMPSITES at Assateague Island National Seashore are not for the faint of heart; they are reached only after a decent walk or paddle and require that you haul in all your gear, even water. Those who do undertake the trip are rewarded with an unparalleled experience—a stunning (and often empty) beach where, on a clear night, accompanied by the soft lap of Atlantic waves, one can gaze into a sky full of stars unimpeded by artificial light. It's like stepping back a century or so, and it offers an unforgettable experience, well worth the work of getting there. You should be aware, however, that unpredictable weather conditions mean that rangers may close off the entire backcountry area; also, you'll have to sign a waiver acknowledging that rescue personnel may not be able to come get you if something goes wrong. Last, you have to be prepared to pack everything in and out; the backcountry of the seashore demands Leave No Trace ethics.

Assateague Island National Seashore has two oceanside backcountry campsites (Little Levels and State Line). Short trails off the beach take you there; it's 4 miles to Little Levels and a haul of 11 miles to the State Line campground. There are also four bayside sites (Tingles Island, Pine Tree, Green Run, and Pope Bay), which can be reached by canoe or kayak. The distances to the bayside campgrounds are more manageable for several reasons: first, obviously, your transport can be your water vessel as opposed to your feet. Second, you have four to choose from instead of just two, which leads to the third reason: shorter distances.

The privacy, spaciousness, and quiet ratings here are averages and depend entirely upon how many people you share the space with, which will be determined mostly by time of year and distance from the headquarters. Rangers issue permits until the maximum

> *While small campsites in forests often lead to a natural inclination to seal yourself within your space, on open beach, with fires roaring, it's almost impossible not to feel that you and your neighbors, here at the end of the earth, are in on something grand.*

RATINGS

Beauty: ✰ ✰ ✰ ✰ ✰
Privacy: ✰ ✰ ✰
Spaciousness: ✰ ✰ ✰ ✰
Quiet: ✰ ✰ ✰ ✰
Security: ✰ ✰ ✰ ✰
Cleanliness: ✰ ✰ ✰ ✰ ✰

number of accommodations for each site fills, so your privacy and space will obviously depend upon the number of people filling the spaces. For individual sites, vacancy is determined by the following formulae: Little Levels and State Line have no limit on the number of groups but max out at 30 and 25 people, respectively (meaning that there may be up to 25 individual campers, or one group of 25, or anything in between). Tingles Island and Pine Tree can have five groups and/or 25 people; Green Run has three groups and/or 15 people, and Pope Bay can have two groups and/or 10 people.

Check-in times vary by site; rangers issue permits based upon the distance one has to travel to get to the site. Based on sunset time, these check-in times will obviously vary over the course of the year. But the following holds steady no matter what time of year: check-in is two hours before sunset for Tingles Island, Little Levels, and Pine Tree; and four hours before sunset for Green Run, State Line, and Pope Bay. Check-in times, as well as distances to campsites and required parking areas, differ if you're coming from Virginia. Visit the AINS Web site for Virginia information and distances.

KEY INFORMATION

ADDRESS:	Assateague Island National Seashore
	7206 National Seashore Lane
	Berlin, MD 21811
	(410) 641-3030
OPERATED BY:	National Park Service
OPEN:	All year, but sites occasionally may be closed due to extreme weather. During spring and summer, one or both backcountry oceanside sites may be closed due to bird nesting. Bayside sites are open all year except briefly during hunting season in autumn (call (410) 641-3030 for hunting dates). Note: The NPS does not recommend camping on the bayside in summer because of the high concentrations of biting insects.
SITES:	6, holding a total maximum of 130 people
EACH SITE HAS:	Picnic tables, fire rings
ASSIGNMENT:	First come, first served
REGISTRATION:	North Beach Ranger Station
FACILITIES:	Chemical toilets
PARKING:	All vehicles must be left at the North Beach Ranger Station for hikers and the Old Ferry Landing Parking Area or Bayside Picnic Area for paddlers
FEE:	$5/backcountry permit and $10 7-day entrance fee per vehicle
RESTRICTIONS:	*Pets:* Prohibited
	Quiet Hours: 10 p.m.–6 a.m.
	Visitors: Must obtain permits
	Fires: In fire rings at bayside sites. Fires allowed on beach below the high-tide line at oceanside sites; fires should be extinguished with water, not sand
	Alcohol: Not permitted
	Stay Limit: Permits are good for up to 7 days and can be renewed
	Other: No fresh water is available at any backcountry site; haul in your own water. You must camp only at site listed on your permit.

As you can imagine, State Line offers the most solitude, as relatively few people are willing to hike 13 miles with camping equipment. But if you are, your rewards will be plentiful; the Atlantic on your left never ceases being beautiful. Little Levels, because it's closer, is more popular. But even if all space gets filled, something wonderful often happens in places like this. While small campsites in forests often lead to a natural inclination to seal yourself within your space (after all, why did you choose to leave your warm and comfortable bed to sleep in the woods?), on open beach, with fires roaring, it's almost impossible not to feel that you and your neighbors, here at the end of the earth, are in on something grand. Assateague's backcountry spaces may well be the only place where you might feel better having lots of neighbors. Then again, maybe not—and if not, go for the State Line section, where your chance for a multitude of neighbors decreases.

It's important to note that rangers do not recommend summer camping in the bayside sites, which are havens for swarms of biting insects (mosquitoes mostly, but all those horses running around assure some nasty horseflies, too). There's one annoyance to the oceanside sites as well, though it certainly shouldn't deter you: the beach from the Ranger Station to the state line is an Over Sand Vehicle (OSV) zone. Expect to see some trucks churning up and down the beach. These can certainly shatter the harmony of an oceanside hike along the water line, but all the "traffic" will be gone by the time you bed down for the night.

While many oceanside sites offer the attraction of sleeping near the ocean, the bayside sites, aside from Pope Bay, offer forest and shade. While this is an important consideration, your destination should probably depend upon how much paddling you're willing or wanting to do to get there: Tingles Island requires a paddle of 3 miles, Pine Tree is 6 miles, Green Run is 10.5 miles, and Pope Bay is a trip of 14 miles. Tingles Island can be quick and easy, and you'll be on the edge of beautiful Tingles Narrows, studded with little islands that hum with birdsong. Pine Tree requires you to pass through Tingles Narrows before an easy take-out at the campsite. Green Run sits at the tip of Green Run Bay, a cove just beyond the Pirate Islands. Last is Pope Bay, which sits in the bay of the same name and is really a wonderful kayak trip. Getting there requires weaving through lots of marshland alive with waterfowl—well worth the strenuous trip. In the case of these bayside backcountry sites, getting there can be half the fun.

MAP

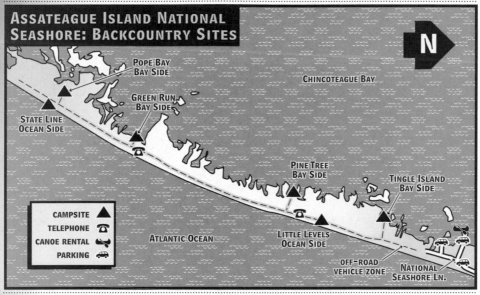

ASSATEAGUE ISLAND NATIONAL SEASHORE: BACKCOUNTRY SITES

POPE BAY
BAY SIDE

GREEN RUN
BAY SIDE

STATE LINE
OCEAN SIDE

CHINCOTEAGUE BAY

PINE TREE
BAY SIDE

TINGLE ISLAND
BAY SIDE

CAMPSITE
TELEPHONE
CANOE RENTAL
PARKING

ATLANTIC OCEAN

LITTLE LEVELS
OCEAN SIDE

OFF-ROAD
VEHICLE ZONE

NATIONAL
SEASHORE LN.

GETTING THERE

Take US Route 50 just
before Ocean City to
MD 611 South.

GPS COORDINATES

UTM Zone (NAD27) 18S
Easting 485444
Northing 4225007

NOT TO BE CONFUSED WITH Assateague Island National Seashore, Assateague State Park is run by the Maryland Department of Natural Resources. In what's an oft-quoted boast, *National Geographic Traveler* selected Assateague State Park as one of the ten best state parks in America in 1994. While the boast has begun to feel a bit dated, the park still lives up to that lofty standard. Assateague State Park is the only ocean park in the state parks system, hemmed in by the Atlantic on one side and Sinepuxent Bay on the other, located on Assateague Island.

At one time in the not so distant past, the camp loops were being eaten away by shifting sand dunes. At the beginning of the 1990s, the dunes stood at almost 20 feet above sea level. But big storms wiped out the dunes by the end of the decade. Recent restoration has put the dunes back in place. Some people have complained about this, as the view from the campsites used to be of the ocean. Now the ocean sits behind walls of sand. But the dunes are integral to protecting the island, just as the island is integral to protecting the mainland.

Owing to its popularity, Assateague State Park has some 350 campsites spread over ten loops (A to J). Don't expect to have the place to yourself. Worse, in summer you'd be willing to trade the mosquitoes for another thousand people. Still, a book on Maryland camping must include Assateague. Simply put, it's a special place. Deer and wild ponies wander the area like animals used to human contact (which, of course, they are). This can create some problems, such as when they are unwilling to leave your campsite or get out of the way of your car. There are strict policies against feeding or touching any animals.

Loop A has 22 sites and a bathhouse. Sites 10 to 15 are closest to the ocean. I must note, however, that

> National Geographic Traveler *selected Assateague State Park as one of the ten best state parks in America.*

RATINGS

Beauty: ☆ ☆ ☆ ☆ ☆
Privacy: ☆ ☆ ☆
Spaciousness: ☆ ☆ ☆
Quiet: ☆ ☆ ☆
Security: ☆ ☆ ☆ ☆ ☆
Cleanliness: ☆ ☆ ☆ ☆

KEY INFORMATION

"closest to the ocean" means some 40 yards or so—nothing too terrible, but this is true of all the camp loops. Sites 1, 2, 21, and 22 are nearest the main camp road, Ocean Drive. All the sites are decent size, but if you require room, the biggest in Loop A are 2 and 22, both of which sit on the internal loop immediately after entering from Ocean Drive.

Loop B has 24 sites. Sites 9 to 15 are closest to the ocean, and 1, 2, 23, and 24 are nearest Ocean Drive. B shares a bathhouse with Loop C. The two largest sites in B are 22 and 12.

Loop C has 24 sites. Sites 12 and 13 are closest to the ocean, and 1, 2, 23, and 24 are nearest Ocean Drive. The largest sites are 13 and 20. Site 13 also sits on the northeastern corner of the loop road, nearest the ocean, so it's a nice spot.

Loop D has 28 sites, and a bathhouse, and sits adjacent to the nature center. Sites 14 to 17 are closest to the beach, and 1, 2, 27, and 28 are nearest Ocean Drive. Sites 13 to 17 are smaller than the rest, which look to be pretty uniform in size.

Loops E to G have sites that are generally larger than those found in A to D. Loop E contains a bathhouse (sites 14 to 18 are closest to the ocean, and 1, 2, 3, and 30 are nearest Ocean Drive); Loop F has a bathhouse and 30 sites. Sites 4, 6, 9, and 10 are wheelchair accessible (sites 15 to 19 are closest to the ocean, and 1 and 2 are near Ocean Drive); Loop G has 30 sites (sites 14 to 17 are closest to the ocean, and 1, 2, and 30 are nearest Ocean Drive; additionally, sites 7 to 11 sit near a bathhouse and a dumping station); Loop H has 39 sites, all of them electric, so if tent camping, skip Loop H. Loop I has two bathhouses and an astounding, tightly packed 110 sites. The sites aren't very much smaller than those in E to G, but there are just so many folks with whom you have to share the loop.

In my opinion, the best option is Loop J, the southernmost loop. No one else will be driving past your campsite, as J is the end and contains only 13 sites, as well as a bathhouse. Sites 11, 12, and 13 may very well be the best in the entire park because they sit closest to the ocean. The sites here are a little smaller than elsewhere in the park, but there's certainly room

MAP

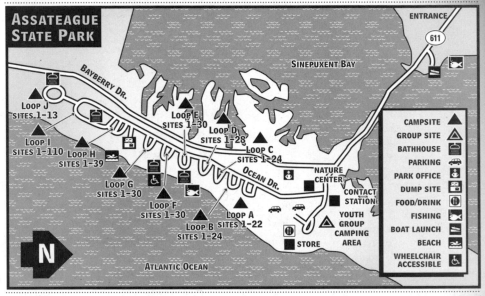

ASSATEAGUE STATE PARK

ENTRANCE

611

SINEPUXENT BAY

BAYBERRY DR.

LOOP J
SITES 1-13

LOOP E
SITES 1-30

LOOP D
SITES 1-28

LOOP C
SITES 1-24

LOOP I
SITES 1-110

LOOP H
SITES 1-39

OCEAN DR.

NATURE
CENTER

LOOP G
SITES 1-30

CONTACT
STATION

LOOP F
SITES 1-30

LOOP A
SITES 1-22

YOUTH
GROUP
CAMPING
AREA

LOOP B
SITES 1-24

STORE

N

ATLANTIC OCEAN

CAMPSITE
GROUP SITE
BATHHOUSE
PARKING
PARK OFFICE
DUMP SITE
FOOD/DRINK
FISHING
BOAT LAUNCH
BEACH
WHEELCHAIR
ACCESSIBLE

enough, and what you give up in space is worth it.

With so many spots, it's difficult to recommend many specific ones. It might be best to consult the campground map and make your decision based upon your particular wants and needs, such as proximity to bathhouses or ocean. There is one last consideration to help guide you. For the sandiest spots, which many people find attractive because they give the best sense of the ocean, head to Loop A. If you prefer more vegetation, which provides the advantage of potential shade, go for Loop E or F.

GETTING THERE

Take US 50 to MD Route 611, 8 miles south of Ocean City.

GPS COORDINATES

UTM Zone (NAD27) 18S
Easting 487860
Northing 4231855

> *Picture-perfect tidewater Maryland.*

JANES ISLAND STATE PARK, at 3,147 acres, is thought of in two parts: the developed section and the outlying, rugged area accessible only by boat. And in between? Picture-perfect tidewater Maryland. As an added bonus, thousands of migrating waterfowl that stop over at nearby Blackwater National Wildlife Refuge can be easily spotted in and around Janes Island. It is, in a word, beautiful.

America's history is inextricably linked with Maryland's, and that may be truer of the area around Janes Island than anywhere else. Settled in 1658 by English colonists, it was first explored by John Smith the year after Jamestown was settled. Smith, no doubt, came upon the original inhabitants, Annemessex Native Americans. To this day, Annemessex artifacts can be found at close by Smith Island's shores. From nearby Crisfield, the "end of the land," you can get a ferry to Smith Island, the no-stoplight place where, purportedly, the locals speak the New World's closest thing to English. (I must admit, the local twang doesn't sound very British to me.) Indeed, many of the island's residents can trace their lineage to those first English settlers.

Janes Island has been designated part of the Chesapeake Bay Gateway, a series of parks, wildlife refuges, museums, ships, historic communities, and trails—"special places where you can experience the authentic Chesapeake." Janes Island is also part of the Beach to Bay Indian Trail, stretching 55 miles from the Atlantic to the Bay, roughly following Native American trails.

This is a water park, dominated by Tangier Sound to the west and the Big Annemessex River to the north. Accordingly, Janes Island offers six water trails: Red, Brown, Yellow, Green, Black, and Blue. Each offers unique access to area waterways; the Blue Trail, for

RATINGS

Beauty: ✿ ✿ ✿ ✿ ✿
Privacy: ✿ ✿ ✿ ✿
Spaciousness: ✿ ✿ ✿
Quiet: ✿ ✿ ✿ ✿
Security: ✿ ✿ ✿ ✿ ✿
Cleanliness: ✿ ✿ ✿ ✿

instance, takes in Ward Creek, the Daugherty Creek Canal, and the Little Annemessex River. The Black, Blue, Red, and Yellow trails all wind through the creeks and marshland within the island. The Green and Brown trails head all the way out to Tangier Sound and are for experienced paddlers. With all these options, you'll be satisfied no matter what your skill level.

You enter the park on Alfred J. Lawson Drive and head straight toward Daugherty Creek Canal, which gives access to the water trails. Loop A is the closest to all the action: the marina, boat launch, bathhouse, trailer storage, etc. No matter where you stay in the campground, you'll come this way when it's time to launch. Loop A contains sites 41 to 66. Sites 47 to 51 are actually the most pleasant if what you're looking for is space from your neighbors; however, they are all electric.

Loop B contains sites 1 to 40. It's relatively small and tucked up toward the canal from the roads leading to and from Loop A and C. This is Janes Island's electric loop, so skip it in favor of Loop C, which is entirely nonelectric.

Loop C (70 to 104) contains the park's best sites. Because of their nonelectric status and proximity to the water, the best of the best are sites 74 to79, which sit on the outside loop near Daugherty Creek Canal. My favorite in the park, however, is Site 81, which also sits by the water but does not have the loop road in between and sits more by itself than the others, providing your best bet for privacy.

There is one last camping option at Janes Island State Park. There are three primitive sites in the park: one on the north side, one on the south side, and one in the middle of the island. Each is accessible only by canoe or kayak and requires you to pack out everything. One word of warning if this roughing it appeals to you: the mosquitoes are worse here than in the campground (if that can be believed). The permits for the primitive sites cost $7 and can be obtained at the camp store.

KEY INFORMATION

ADDRESS:	**Janes Island S. P. 26280 Alfred J. Lawson Drive Crisfield, MD 21817 (410) 968-1565**
OPERATED BY:	**Maryland Department of Natural Resources**
OPEN:	**Last weekend in April–October**
SITES:	**104**
EACH SITE HAS:	**Picnic table, fire ring**
ASSIGNMENT:	**Reservations recommended**
REGISTRATION:	**(888) 432-CAMP (2267) or at http:// reservations .dnr.state.md.us**
FACILITIES:	**Boat launch and rental, camp store, conference center, dump station, playground, visitor center**
PARKING:	**At designated spots**
FEE:	**$25/night, $30/night electric; boat launch, $7/vehicle; out-of-state residents, $8/vehicle**
RESTRICTIONS:	*Pets:* **Not allowed** *Quiet Hours:* **11 p.m.–7 a.m.** *Visitors:* **Must register if staying overnight, otherwise must leave by 11 p.m.** *Fires:* **No open fires** *Alcohol:* **Permitted** *Stay Limit:* **None** *Other:* **Mosquitoes are serious business at Janes Island. Camping here without defense can ruin your stay. Try The Defender, from Burt's Bees.**

MAP

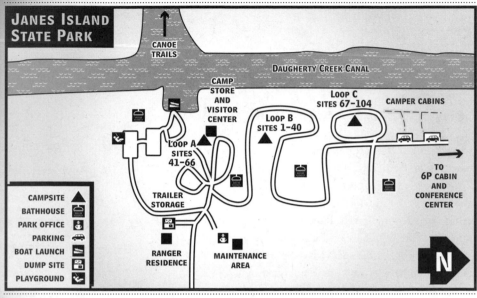

JANES ISLAND STATE PARK

CANOE TRAILS

DAUGHERTY CREEK CANAL

CAMP STORE AND VISITOR CENTER

LOOP C SITES 67–104

CAMPER CABINS

LOOP B SITES 1–40

LOOP A SITES 41–66

TO 6P CABIN AND CONFERENCE CENTER

TRAILER STORAGE

RANGER RESIDENCE

MAINTENANCE AREA

CAMPSITE
BATHHOUSE
PARK OFFICE
PARKING
BOAT LAUNCH
DUMP SITE
PLAYGROUND

N

GETTING THERE

Take MD Route 13 to Westover. Take MD Route 413 south, approximately 11 miles to a right on Plantation Road (which becomes Jacksonville Road), and take a right onto Alfred Lawson Drive.

GPS COORDINATES

UTM Zone (NAD27) 18S
Easting 425665
Northing 4207468

MARTINAK STATE PARK

ON THE SITE OF A FORMER INDIAN VILLAGE, Martinak State Park is small at only 107 acres, but that's partly because it's hemmed in by so much water. Bordered by the Choptank River (the Chesapeake's largest Eastern Shore tributary) and Watts Creek, Martinak is understandably popular as a fishing and boating haven. Bass, catfish, perch, and sunfish are the popular catches in and around the park (you must have a Chesapeake Bay Sportfishing License). Both waterways are surrounded by hardwood and pine forests, providing great hiking and birding as well. A birding camp in July and a bass-fishing camp in August will teach you how to increase your chances in both.

Other special programs also make Martinak very family friendly. A youth fishing derby, a junior ranger program, and "Summer Park Pals" for 4-to-6 year-olds are just some of Martinak State Park's special events. Summer concerts and country auctions also pull people from all over the Eastern Shore. While the crowds these events attract might turn some people off, Martinak always feels like a friendly and pleasant place to be. In fact, most campers you'll meet at Martinak are folks who return year after year, giving the place a very fraternal feel.

At a time when many state and national parks are scaling back activities because of severe budget limitations, Martinak has seen a recent upgrade in many of its facilities, as well as the addition of new trails and walkways. Part of this largesse comes from the spoils of Martinak's status as a Chesapeake Bay Gateway in a system coordinated by the National Park Service that designates Chesapeake watershed properties as worthy of protection and educational outreach. Improvements to Martinak's nature center, for example, come in part from the Gateways Network. Now, a library, aquarium,

> *Martinak has seen a recent upgrade in many of its facilities, as well as the addition of new trails and walkways.*

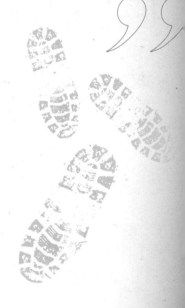

RATINGS

Beauty: ✰ ✰ ✰ ✰
Privacy: ✰ ✰ ✰ ✰
Spaciousness: ✰ ✰ ✰
Quiet: ✰ ✰ ✰ ✰
Security: ✰ ✰ ✰ ✰ ✰
Cleanliness: ✰ ✰ ✰ ✰

KEY INFORMATION

ADDRESS: **Martinak State Park
137 Deep Shore
Road
Denton, MD 21629
(410) 820-1668**

OPERATED BY: **Maryland Department of Natural
Resources**

OPEN: **End of March–
October**

SITES: **63**

EACH SITE HAS: **Camping pad, picnic
table, fire ring**

ASSIGNMENT: **Reservations
recommended for
holiday weekends**

REGISTRATION: **(888) 432-CAMP
(2267) or http://
reservations.dnr
.state.md.us**

FACILITIES: **Bathhouse, dump
station, boat launch,
playground, shelters,
nature center**

PARKING: **In designated spots**

FEE: **$20/night, $25/night
electric**

RESTRICTIONS: *Pets:* **Allowed on
leash**
Quiet Hours: **11 p.m.–
7 a.m.**
Visitors: **Register
at campground
entrance**
Fires: **In fire rings**
Alcohol: **Permitted at
site**
Stay Limit: **2 weeks**

and live and stuffed animals are just part of what's to see in the nature center.

There are two camping loops (A and B) in Martinak. Loop A has 30 sites (plus four camper cabins), reservable for either tents or RVs, so who you get as a neighbor is something of a crapshoot. All sites sit on the outer loop; aside from the four camper cabins across from sites 16 to 21, there is no other camping inside the loop. The sites on the southern end of the loop (7 to 12) offer the most space between you and your neighbors. A hiking trail, which begins and terminates at Deep Shore Road, completely encircles the camp loop. It's easy to access the trail from anywhere in the camp loop.

Loop B has virtually the same setup as A, with playground equipment and a bathhouse in the middle of the loop. The only significant difference is your choice of three tent-only sites (T-1, T-2, and T-3), but they are nearest the entrance road as well as the dumpster down the street. Like Tuckahoe State Park (see page 164), which is administered by the same central office, the sites at Martinak are pretty uniform. They are all in nicely treed areas and have a good amount of space between them. The truth is, much thoughtfulness went into creating these sites; they are all pretty good and should provide for a pleasant experience.

MAP

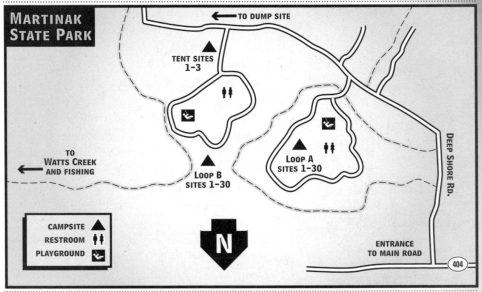

MARTINAK STATE PARK

← TO DUMP SITE

TENT SITES
1-3

TO
WATTS CREEK
AND FISHING ←

LOOP B
SITES 1-30

LOOP A
SITES 1-30

DEEP SHORE RD.

ENTRANCE
TO MAIN ROAD

404

N

CAMPSITE
RESTROOM
PLAYGROUND

GETTING THERE

Take MD Route 404 south of
Denton and turn right on
Deep Shore Road.

GPS COORDINATES

UTM Zone (NAD27) 18S
Easting 427407
Northing 4301954

> *Most Marylanders would be surprised to learn that 12 species of orchid grow in their state—and they can all be found here.*

POCOMOKE RIVER STATE PARK and Forest is glorious, a nature-lover's paradise. It's no secret, however—it got billing in the November 2006 issue of *National Geographic Adventure*. Pocomoke River State Park has two developed areas: Milburn Landing and Shad Landing. They both sit on the Pocomoke River, on opposite sides of the Pocomoke Cypress Swamp. Water access shouldn't necessarily be the thing that determines which of the two areas is your destination. In fact, you can paddle from one to the other (though established water trails are more abundant at Shad Landing. So Shad is arguably the better spot if your primary interest is boating.) But if it's hiking you're after, Milburn allows slightly quicker forest access to almost 15,000 acres of wooded forest. The park's signature feature is the cypress swamps filled with the dark water of the Pocomoke River ("Pocomoke" actually means "black water" in Algonquin.) The Nature Conservancy owns the adjacent Nassawango Creek Preserve, which runs 9,300 acres and hosts, among other must-see wildlife, some 20 species of neotropical migratory birds.

Well-marked canoe trails are easy to follow as they wind through the swamp and tributary rivers and streams. The park is set up mostly for boaters, and for good reason. Canoeing through the 30-mile Pocomoke River Swamp is a primordial experience, one that most people associate with more southern locales. In fact, Pocomoke's swamp is the northernmost example of southern cypress swamps still surviving. Most Marylanders would be surprised to learn that 12 species of orchid grows in their state—and they can all be found here. It is thought also that the swamp provided a safe haven for runaway slaves during the Civil War, as well as pirates and bootleggers. If fishing is your thing, the park's waters boast more than 50 fish species.

RATINGS

Beauty: ✫ ✫ ✫ ✫ ✫
Privacy: ✫ ✫ ✫ ✫
Spaciousness: ✫ ✫ ✫
Quiet: ✫ ✫ ✫ ✫
Security: ✫ ✫ ✫ ✫ ✫
Cleanliness: ✫ ✫ ✫ ✫ ✫

Those wishing for great hiking shouldn't turn away from Pocomoke. Many acres of upland forest, full of loblolly pines and spring wildflowers, offer the trekker much. On a waterside hike here, I saw loads of river otters, a great sight coming right on the heels of watching wheeling herons and eagles.

The Milburn Landing Area is much smaller than the Shad Landing Area, with 36 sites total. It's also a bit cheaper than Shad, but the difference is only $5, so don't let that determine where you stay. Better determinants include number of facilities (Shad has much more infrastructure) and number of people (Shad has much more of that, too). Pet concerns factor in, too. If you've got one, Milburn has to be your destination, as Shad doesn't allow them. In short, if you desire more of a roughing-it feel without the threat of large crowds, Milburn should be your choice. If you want winter camping, which also guarantees small numbers of people, head to Shad, as Milburn closes by mid-December. If you need more facilities, especially if you've got the kids with you, Shad is probably the better choice.

Ecologically, there's not much difference between the two; both offer all the natural attractions provided by the river, forest, streams, and swamp. And it's only a 20-minute drive between the two sites anyway.

Coming in off the Main Road and passing both the boat launch and the Camper Registration Office, you'll head around the dump station and the road to the state forest before coming to the campground. Sites 1 to 15 sit huddled along the first camp road, before coming to the well-spaced and more isolated sites 16 and 17. Sites 18 to 29 are next, located diagonally across from one another along the camp road. When I visited Milburn, it was during drought conditions and I specifically made notes suggesting that the prized camping spots are 34, 35, and 36 because they are closest to the river. However, a subsequent conversation with a ranger clued me into something I would have missed. Because of poor soil conditions, these three sites can be wet and are plagued with persistent drainage problems. If it rains during your stay, this can be a real downer, obviously. This same ranger suggested sites 1 to 22. They sit right under the trees, with no stone dust pad. Sites 18 to

KEY INFORMATION

ADDRESS: Pocomoke River State Park 3461 Worcester Highway Snow Hill, MD 21863 (410) 632-2566

OPERATED BY: Maryland Department of Natural Resources

OPEN: Last weekend in April–mid-December; camping during weekends only last weekend in September–the end of season

SITES: 36 total (4 mini-cabins)

EACH SITE HAS: Picnic table, fire ring

ASSIGNMENT: Self-register at Camper Registration Office

REGISTRATION: (888) 432-CAMP (2267), at http://reservations/dnr.state.md.us, or on site

FACILITIES: Bathhouse, boat launch, dump station

PARKING: In designated spots

FEE: $20/night, $25/night electric

RESTRICTIONS: *Pets:* Permitted *Quiet Hours:* 11 p.m.–7 a.m. *Visitors:* Must register at registration station *Fires:* In fire rings *Alcohol:* Permitted at sites *Stay Limit:* 2 weeks, can come back after 1 week away *Other:* Check-out 3 p.m.

MAP

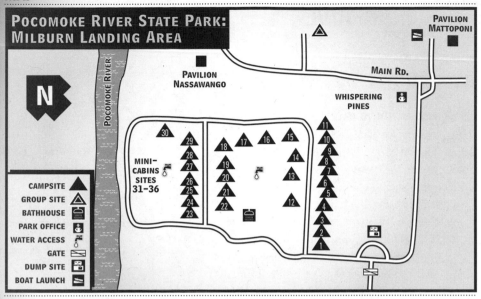

POCOMOKE RIVER STATE PARK: MILBURN LANDING AREA

PAVILION MATTOPONI

MAIN RD.

PAVILION NASSAWANGO

WHISPERING PINES

MINI-CABINS SITES 31–36

| CAMPSITE |
| GROUP SITE |
| BATHHOUSE |
| PARK OFFICE |
| WATER ACCESS |
| GATE |
| DUMP SITE |
| BOAT LAUNCH |

POCOMOKE RIVER

GETTING THERE

Take MD Route 13 South from Salisbury to MD Route 364 East.

22 are inside the road, closer to the bathhouse, but a bit farther from the river than 23 to 29 and especially 34 to 36 (30 to 33 are cabins).

GPS COORDINATES

UTM Zone (NAD27) 18S
Easting 462682
Northing 4221937

SHAD **LANDING IS BY FAR** the busier of Pocomoke State Park's two developed areas. It also offers much more in the way of facilities. Shad Landing feels very much like what you'd expect from a campground offering such amenities and natural attractions: busy. But it does manage to remain relatively laid-back. I think it's the splendor of the area that makes people slow down and take stock.

Aside from the multitude of facilities and the abundance of campsites, two water trails distinguish Shad Landing from the smaller Milburn Landing. Because Shad Landing's campground is bordered both by the Pocomoke River and Corkers Creek, the Corkers Creek Blackwater Canoe Trail, taking in the best of the cypress swamp, is easy to access. But the granddaddy water trail is the one from Shad Landing to Porter's Crossing. This 11-mile water trail is not for the novice. It heads upriver on the Pocomoke and past Snow Hill to a remote area where civilization melts away. Of course, it's possible to access these trails from Milburn, but the 4.5-mile trip required to get just to Shad makes the trip to Porter's Landing prohibitive for novices.

The Shad Landing area has six loops: Fox Den (A), Deer Run (B), Robin's Nest (D), Blue Heron (E), Water's Edge (F), and Acorn Trail (G), plus a youth camping area. Shad Landing is bounded by the Pocomoke River to the west, Corkers Creek to the south, and Route 113 to the east.

Acorn Trail is the northernmost loop and has 30 sites, all electric, so if you're in a tent, you'd do best to avoid it. It's also closest to the busy boat launch. Water's Edge isn't misnamed—it sits the closest to the Pocomoke and is thus among the first to fill up. It has 30 sites. The boardwalk separates the river from sites 87 and 88. It too can get quite busy, so being so near

> *The water trail from Shad Landing to Porter's Crossing heads upriver on the Pocomoke and past Snow Hill to a remote area where civilization melts away.*

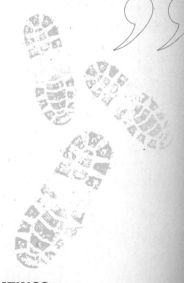

RATINGS

Beauty: ☆ ☆ ☆ ☆
Privacy: ☆ ☆ ☆ ☆
Spaciousness: ☆ ☆ ☆
Quiet: ☆ ☆ ☆ ☆
Security: ☆ ☆ ☆ ☆ ☆
Cleanliness: ☆ ☆ ☆ ☆ ☆

ADDRESS: Pocomoke River State Forest/Park
3461 Worcester Highway
Snow Hill, MD 21863
(410) 632-2566

OPERATED BY: Maryland Department of Natural Resources

OPEN: End of March–September; Robins Nest (171–200) and Waters Edge (61–88) loops open all year for primitive camping

SITES: 200 (8 cabins)

EACH SITE HAS: Picnic table, fire ring

ASSIGNMENT: Reservations recommended

REGISTRATION: (888) 432-2267 or http://reservations.dnr.state.md.us

FACILITIES: Boat launch and rental, camp store, dump station, concessions, electrical hook-ups, picnic areas and shelters, playgrounds, picnic shelters, swimming pool, visitor center

PARKING: In designated spots

FEE: $25/night; $30/night electric

RESTRICTIONS: *Pets:* Not permitted
Quiet Hours: 11 p.m.–7 a.m.
Fires: In fire rings
Alcohol: Permitted at sites
Stay Limit: 2 weeks, can come back after 1 week away
Other: Check-out 3 p.m.

the water might not be as desirable as you might assume. Still, Water's Edge remains understandably popular, especially with tent campers. There's also a marina parking lot near sites 88 and 85. My recommendation is to try for Site 86, which has nothing between it and the water and is sufficiently far away from the boardwalk and marina.

Fox Den also has 30 sites running in a loop, with a bathhouse in the middle. Many people try to avoid sites 40 and 41 on the south end of the loop and 51 to 54 on the north end because a power-line cut runs between them. However, people often fail to consider the nighttime view afforded by clearings. On a clear night, you might just be happy to be near a power line. Deer Run, the next site south of Fox Den, has 30 electric sites; avoid it if you're in a tent.

Robin's Nest seems to be a hub of activity and can get busy, with nearby ball fields and playgrounds. Additionally, the loop contains eight cabins, which can throw light and noise. However, Robin's Nest offers Shad Landing's only wheelchair-accessible camping (sites 183, 185, 195, and 200). The Blue Heron Loop has no developed pads and is more appropriate for tent camping. This was confirmed by a park ranger I spoke to, who suggested that the best loops for tent campers are Blue Heron and Water's Edge. These sites offer pad-free camping, which gives a better outdoorsy feel. Another bonus of the Blue Heron Loop is that its southern edge sits close to Corkers Creek. If you wish to be closest to the water, your best bets are sites 124, 129, 135, 141, or 151.

MAP

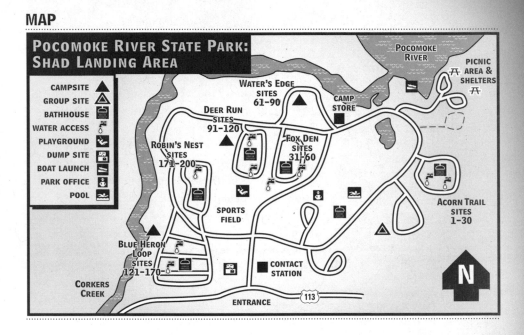

GPS COORDINATES

UTM Zone (NAD27) 18S

Easting 461327

Northing 4220634

48
POINT LOOKOUT
STATE PARK

> *Between the camping,*
> *the swimming, the*
> *scenery, and the*
> *history, you can keep*
> *yourself joyfully*
> *occupied for days.*

POINT LOOKOUT IS ALL ABOUT the water. The entire park and campgrounds are surrounded: Lake Conoy and Point Lookout Creek split the peninsula, while the Potomac River and Chesapeake Bay meet at the southern edge. It's an exceedingly beautiful spot, though its history tells a darker tale. A Civil War prison camp on the site once housed more than 50,000 Confederate troops. Now, the place couldn't be more peaceful.

If you want hiking, you may be disappointed. The Periwinkle Point Trail (less than a mile in length) is the park's only land trail (though you can connect the park's paved roads for a hike of about 5 miles). The abundance of water and tidal action make land trails superfluous. But if you've brought the kayak or canoe, this place is paradise. Three distinct water trails lead you in and around the park: Green Points (1.7 miles) along the Lake Conoy shoreline; Heron Alley Trail (3.4 miles) through Point Lookout Creek; and Lighthouse Trail (3 miles), through tough wind-whipped open water over and around Civil War sites. Each trail can be taken as a day's highlight, or they can be merged and repeated; they never get old.

If you don't have a water vessel, you need not cross off Point Lookout and avoid it altogether. Between the camping, the swimming, the scenery, and the history, you can keep yourself joyfully occupied for days. There are six camp loops, hemmed in by Lake Conoy, Point Lookout Creek, and Tanner's Creek. Most of the recreational activities and infrastructure at Point Lookout State Park are congregated toward the south of the campground, near the confluence of the Potomac and the Chesapeake. Contact stations, Route 5, and dumping and electric hook-up stations for RVs are all near the campground. Nevertheless, the sites are

RATINGS

Beauty: ✪ ✪ ✪ ✪ ✪
Privacy: ✪ ✪ ✪
Spaciousness: ✪ ✪ ✪
Quiet: ✪ ✪ ✪
Security: ✪ ✪ ✪ ✪ ✪
Cleanliness: ✪ ✪ ✪ ✪

fairly well spaced, large, and some are very wooded. Despite the nearby activity, the place manages to feel relaxed and roomy.

The Tulip Loop (F) is the northernmost and sits not too far from the road, especially sites 76 to 80. That said, it's heavily forested and many sites can feel quite remote when the sun goes down. A knock against site 80 is its proximity to electrical hook-ups for RVs. Sites 82, 83, and those on the western side of the Tulip Loop's entrance lane are the preferable ones.

The Malone Loop (E) and Green's Point Loop (B) allow leashed pets. Green's Point sits nearest Lake Conoy, which makes it the park's most popular loop, astride the small youth camping site (Conoy Loop [C], with six cabins). However, Green's has full hook-ups, so it's probably best avoided. If you do find yourself here, sites 100 to 105 sit nearest the pier and have the best water access. Additionally, two wheelchair-accessible sites, 92 and 106, are available. As for Malone Loop, the sites on the outer edge (44 to 52) offer easy access to Point Lookout's one nature trail, short but pleasant.

Lanier Loop (D) contains 26 sites; the southwestern ones abut overflow parking and are also near the visitor center. Sites 3 to 15 offer the most privacy.

KEY INFORMATION

ADDRESS: 11175 Point Lookout Road
Scotland, MD 20687
(301) 872-5688

OPERATED BY: Maryland Department of Natural Resources

OPEN: First weekend in April–late October

SITES: 143

EACH SITE HAS: Picnic table, fire ring

ASSIGNMENT: At camp office or park headquarters during open hours; self-registration otherwise

REGISTRATION: (888) 432-CAMP (2267), http://reservations.dnr.state.md.us, or at ranger station

FACILITIES: Boat launch, boat rental, camp store, bathhouses, dumping station

PARKING: Each site has space for 2–3 vehicles; overflow parking available

FEE: $25/night, $30/night electric, $35/night water, sewer, and electric; $40–$45/night double sites accommodating 12 guests; day-use service charge: May–September weekends and holidays, $5/person; May–September weekdays and October–April, $3/vehicle; boat launch, $10/vehicle; out-of-state residents add $1 to all service charges

RESTRICTIONS: *Pets:* Leashed pets allowed in Malone Circle, Green's Point Loop, Tulip Loop, Hoffman's Loop
Quiet Hours: 11 p.m.–7 a.m.
Visitors: Must leave campground by 10 p.m.
Fires: In fire ring or grill
Alcohol: Allowed
Stay Limit: 2 weeks, but can return after 24 hours
Other: Max. 6 people (except sites 107 and 128, which allow 12 people); check-in and check-out, 3 p.m.

MAP

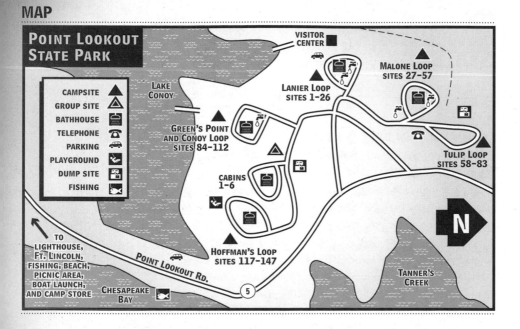

Point Lookout State Park

VISITOR CENTER

MALONE LOOP
SITES 27–57

LAKE CONOY

LANIER LOOP
SITES 1–26

CAMPSITE
GROUP SITE
BATHHOUSE
TELEPHONE
PARKING
PLAYGROUND
DUMP SITE
FISHING

GREEN'S POINT
AND CONOY LOOP
SITES 84–112

TULIP LOOP
SITES 58–83

CABINS
1–6

N

TO
LIGHTHOUSE,
FT. LINCOLN,
FISHING, BEACH,
PICNIC AREA,
BOAT LAUNCH,
AND CAMP STORE

HOFFMAN'S LOOP
SITES 117–147

POINT LOOKOUT RD.

TANNER'S
CREEK

CHESAPEAKE
BAY

5

GETTING THERE

Take US Route 301 to MD Route 4 South in Upper Marlboro. Follow Route 4 across the Solomons Island Bridge. Turn left onto MD Route 235 South. Turn left onto MD Route 5 South to the park (7 miles).

The final loop, Hoffman's (A), offers 31 sites, including two wheelchair-accessible sites, 123 and 140. The closest to Route 5 are sites 135 to 144, while 122 to 131 promise Hoffman's more private spots. Hoffman's is tent-only and is close to the water, so I would highly recommend it.

Again, Point Lookout has a lot of spots in a relatively small space, typical of such popular family campgrounds. This doesn't mean you won't have a pleasant experience. Again, if you've brought the boat, and especially if it's off-season, the beauty of the area and the wonderful water trails never fail to impress and inspire.

GPS COORDINATES

UTM Zone (NAD27) 18S
Easting 382455
Northing 4214299

49
SMALLWOOD
STATE PARK

SMALLWOOD STATE PARK TAKES its name from its prominent early resident, Revolutionary War General William Smallwood, later Maryland's fourth governor. His house, Smallwood's Retreat, sits on park property and can be visited from 1 to 5 p.m. on Sundays. Tours are conducted by costumed docents.

Smallwood State Park is a relatively small park, at 630 acres. However, it looms large in its year-round status as Maryland's premier host for bass-fishing tournaments. Record fish are frequently pulled from the Potomac at Smallwood State Park. Even if you're not interested in a tournament, the fishing here is sublime, and pervasive. You can fish for bass, carp, catfish, hardhead, and perch; a Chesapeake Bay Sportfishing License is required. Hiking trails are minimal—the entire trail system is barely 2 miles.

Along with its history and fishing, another Smallwood attraction is its proximity to Mattawoman Creek, a tributary of the Potomac River. The creek is duly popular with boaters and anglers using Sweden Point Marina—expect large boats and towing trucks and RVs. In fact, all of Smallwood's 15 sites are electric. However, don't let this turn you away from this wonderful diminutive campground. With six launch slips, it's easy to squirm your way in if you have a smaller vessel. Because the campsite is small, it's never crowded (even at capacity), and the vast majority of visitors to Smallwood are day-users. Plus, it's a beautiful spot well worth a visit and not far from D.C.'s eastern suburbs.

Visiting Smallwood State Park will give you the distinct feeling that this is a family getaway. The large recycled-tire playground, with fish theme, plays a large part in that. A nice touch: most of the playground's equipment is wheelchair-accessible. In addition to the restored retreat house, an 18th-century tidewater plantation and 19th-century tobacco barn are also on

> *Smallwood looms large in its year-round status as Maryland's premier host for bass-fishing tournaments.*

RATINGS

Beauty: ✩ ✩ ✩ ✩
Privacy: ✩ ✩ ✩
Spaciousness: ✩ ✩ ✩ ✩ ✩
Quiet: ✩ ✩ ✩ ✩
Security: ✩ ✩ ✩ ✩ ✩
Cleanliness: ✩ ✩ ✩ ✩

the grounds, and interpretive guides help visitors know what life was like back then. Craft demonstrations and military exhibitions are held throughout the year. All of these facts mean that bringing kids along is a great idea.

As stated, all campsites are electric. Additionally, none is terribly far from the next, but each is well shaded under mature hardwoods. Some, by virtue of their large size, can offer at least a modicum of privacy. Sites 12, 2, and 3 are the largest, in that order. Site 1 is also pretty large. Because sites are first come, first served, tent campers can have these large sites if they are available. If you've brought the dog, you're limited to sites 12 to 15. If you detest dogs, stay away by trying to secure one of the lower numbers on the other side of the one-way loop. Sites 3 to 7 (4 to 6 especially) are farthest from the potential activity of the dump station, playground, and footbridge to the marina.

KEY INFORMATION

ADDRESS:	Smallwood State Park
	2750 Sweden Point Road
	Marbury, MD 20658
	(301) 743-7613
OPERATED BY:	Maryland Department of Natural Resources
OPEN:	April–October
SITES:	15, plus 6 camper cabins
EACH SITE HAS:	Picnic table, lantern post, fire ring
ASSIGNMENT:	Campers can register at the Concession Store during the season and at headquarters when the Concession is closed. During the week, a ranger will register you when both facilities are closed. You must check with a ranger prior to setting up in any of the sites.
REGISTRATION:	Recommended between Memorial and Labor Day; (888) 432-CAMP (2267) or http://reservations.dnr.state.md.us
FACILITIES:	Bathhouse, boat launch and rental, dumping station, concessions, marina, picnic shelters, playground
PARKING:	On-site gravel driveway or the nearest marked parking lot; 2 vehicles per site
FEE:	$30/night; April–October weekends and holidays, $3/person $3/vehicle weekdays and remainder of year; boat ramp service charge, $10; out-of-state residents add $1 to all service charges
RESTRICTIONS:	*Pets:* Allowed at sites 12–15
	Quiet Hours: 11 p.m.–7 a.m.
	Visitors: Max. 6 people per site
	Fires: In fire rings
	Alcohol: Permitted
	Stay Limit: 2 weeks; campers can return after 1 week
	Other: Campers must check in by 8:30 p.m.; check-out or renew by 2 p.m.

MAP

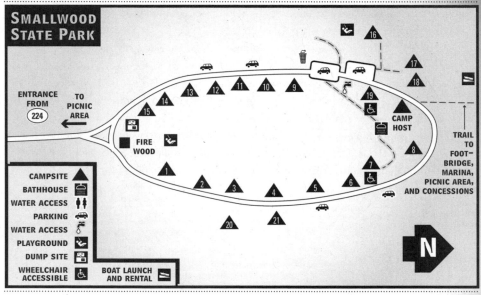

GETTING THERE

Take US Route 301 to La Plata. Go west on MD Route 225 to MD Route 224. At the light at Route 224 turn left (south). Park entrance is approximately 3 miles on the right.

GPS COORDINATES

UTM Zone (NAD27) 18S
Easting 309875
Northing 4269559

50
TUCKAHOE STATE PARK

> *There's something about paddling around trees teeming with herons, ospreys, and bald eagles that feels absolutely primeval.*

TUCKAHOE STATE PARK CONTAINS some indispensable American history. The country's most famous abolitionist, Frederick Douglass, was born along Tuckahoe Creek, and the area also served as part of Harriet Tubman's Underground Railroad. Long before the era of American slavery, the Nanticoke Indians, who appreciated the bounty offered by the creek and surrounding marshland forestlands, inhabited Tuckahoe. Today, the area's natural beauty serves as a stark contrast to its terrible past.

The creek, which serves as the dividing line between Queen Anne's and Caroline counties, bisects the park's 3,800 acres and heads eventually to the Choptank River. Tuckahoe Creek also flows into and out of a 60-acre lake. The park's waterways and forests mean that an almost endless array of recreational opportunities awaits the visitor. Within the park's acreage also lies 500-acre Adkins Arboretum, crisscrossed by 3 miles of hiking trails.

Personally, I think the lake's 40 acres of flooded forestland is the most unique attraction. While the rest of the lake is open water and allows for great fishing, there's something about paddling around trees teeming with herons, ospreys, and bald eagles that feels absolutely primeval. Don't worry if you didn't bring a canoe; the park provides rentals. For a great experience, explore the park's great water trails and then beach to walk more trails (some 15 miles worth in all) throughout the forest.

Another attraction to Tuckahoe is its isolated feel. A perfect jewel of typical Maryland Eastern Shore scenery, it has so far been spared rampant development that threatens so much of the Eastern Shore. In fact, you'll be forgiven if upon first visit you think you've taken a wrong turn and are heading to nowhere, with no infrastructure.

RATINGS

Beauty: ✿ ✿ ✿ ✿
Privacy: ✿ ✿ ✿ ✿
Spaciousness: ✿ ✿ ✿
Quiet: ✿ ✿ ✿
Security: ✿ ✿ ✿ ✿ ✿
Cleanliness: ✿ ✿ ✿ ✿ ✿

There are two camp loops; the electric one sits closer to the lake, while the nonelectric loop sits just north. The electric loop has 34 sites and four cabins. If tent camping, you'll want to choose the nonelectric loop, which is smaller, presents easier access to the canoe launch for Tuckahoe Creek, and offers three tent-only sites (T-1, T-2, T-3). There are only 15 sites total, each with a decent buffer of trees around, plus a bathhouse in the middle. Sites 9 and 10 are nearest the canoe launch and overflow parking. Otherwise, little distinguishes these sites; they are all the same size and sit within a nice copse with sufficient buffer. In short, you can't go wrong with any of them.

KEY INFORMATION

ADDRESS: Tuckahoe State Park
13070 Crouse Mill Road
Queen Anne, MD 21657
(410) 820-1668

OPERATED BY: Maryland Department of Natural Resources

OPEN: Third week of March–October

SITES: 51

EACH SITE HAS: Camping pad, picnic table, fire ring

ASSIGNMENT: Reservations recommend for weekends

REGISTRATION: (888) 432-CAMP (2267) or http://reservations.dnr.state.md.us

FACILITIES: Bathhouse, playground, picnic pavilions, arboretum, boat launch, bike and boat rental

PARKING: In designated spots

FEE: $20/night; $25/night electric

RESTRICTIONS: *Pets:* Allowed on leash
Quiet Hours: 11 p.m.–7 a.m.
Visitors: Register at the campground entrance
Fires: In fire rings
Alcohol: Permitted at site
Stay Limit: 2 weeks
Other: Summertime here means mosquitoes. Be prepared.

MAP

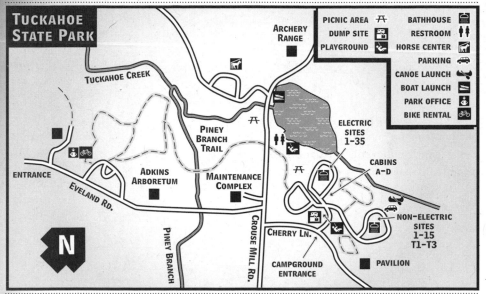

TUCKAHOE STATE PARK

PICNIC AREA
DUMP SITE
PLAYGROUND

BATHHOUSE
RESTROOM
HORSE CENTER
PARKING
CANOE LAUNCH
BOAT LAUNCH
PARK OFFICE
BIKE RENTAL

ARCHERY RANGE

TUCKAHOE CREEK

PINEY BRANCH TRAIL

ELECTRIC SITES 1-35

CABINS A-D

ENTRANCE

ADKINS ARBORETUM

MAINTENANCE COMPLEX

NON-ELECTRIC SITES 1-15 T1-T3

EVELAND RD.

PINEY BRANCH

CROUSE MILL RD.

CHERRY LN.

CAMPGROUND ENTRANCE

PAVILION

N

GETTING THERE

Take US Route 50/301 east of the Bay Bridge. When 50/301 splits, bear to the right on Route 50. Make a left at the intersection of Route 50 and MD Route 404. Go 8 miles until you come to MD Route 480 and take a left. Take first left onto Eveland Road.

GPS COORDINATES

UTM Zone (NAD27) 18S
Easting 418435
Northing 4313629"

APPENDIX & INDEX

CAMPING EQUIPMENT
CHECKLIST

Except for the large and bulky items on this list, I keep a plastic storage container full of the essentials for car camping so they're ready to go when I am. I make a last-minute check of the inventory, resupply anything that's low or missing, and away I go

COOKING UTENSILS

Aluminum foil
Bottle opener
Bottles of salt, pepper, spices, sugar, cooking oil, and maple syrup in waterproof, spillproof containers
Can opener
Corkscrew
Cups, plastic or tin
Dish soap (biodegradable), sponge, and towel
Flatware
Food of your choice
Frying pan
Fuel for stove
Matches in waterproof container
Plates
Pocketknife
Pot with lid
Spatula
Stove
Wooden spoon

FIRST–AID KIT

Antibiotic cream
Band-Aids®
Diphenhydramine (Benadryl®)
Gauze pads
Ibuprofen or aspirin
Insect repellent
Lip balm
Moleskin®
Snakebite kit
Sunscreen
Tape, waterproof adhesive

SLEEPING GEAR

Pillow
Sleeping bag
Sleeping pad, inflatable or insulated
Tent with ground tarp and rainfly

MISCELLANEOUS

Bath soap (biodegradable), washcloth, and towel
Camp chair
Candles
Cooler
Deck of cards
Duct tape
Fire starter
Flashlight or headlamp with fresh batteries
Foul-weather clothing
Paper towels
Plastic zip-top bags
Sunglasses
Toilet paper
Water bottle
Wool or fleece blanket
Optional:
Barbecue grill
Binoculars
Field guides on bird, plant, and wildlife identification
Fishing rod and tackle
Hatchet
Kayak and related paddling gear
Lantern
Maps (road, topographic, trails, and so on)
Mountain bike and related riding gear

INDEX

Addison Run, Cunningham Falls State Park, 34–35
Adkins Arboretum, 164–66
Alcohol regulations. *See specific campgrounds,* key information
Animals, hazardous, 4–5
Annapolis Rock, 63–65, 91–93
Annemessex River, 146–48
Antietam Creek, C&O Canal, 19–22
Antietam National Battlefield, 19–22, 26, 66–68
Appalachian Trail
    Greenbrier State Park, 63–65
    Maple Tree Camp, 66–68
    South Mountain State Park, 87–90, 91–93
Arboretums, 164–66
Archaeologic sites, Janes Island State Park, 146–48
Assateague Island National Seashore
    backcountry sites, 139–42
    Bayside Campground, 134–136
    Oceanside Campground, 136–38
Assateague State Park, 143–45
Atlantic Ocean
Assateague Island National Seashore, 136–38, 139–42
Assateague State Park, 143–45

Back River, Hart Miller Island, 114–16
Backbone Mountain, 48–50, 72–74, 75–77
Backcountry sites
    Assateague Island National Seashore, 139–42
    Garrett State Forest, 51–53
    Potomac State Forest, 72–74
    Savage River State Forest, 84–86
    South Mountain State Park, 91–93
Bald Eagle Island, C&O Canal, 26
Bartman's Hill Trail, Greenbrier State Park, 63–65
Basketball court, Brunswick Family Campground, 13–15
Bayside Campground, Assateague Island National Seashore, 134–36
Beach to Bay Indian Trail, Janes Island State Park, 146–48
Beaches
    Assateague Island National Seashore
        backcountry sites, 139–42
        Bayside Campground, 134–36
        Oceanside Campground, 136–38
    Assateague State Park, 143–45
    Elk Neck State Park, 108–10
    Hart-Miller Island, 114–16
    Janes Island State Park, 146–48

Bear Branch, Cunningham Falls State Park, 34–35
Berlin
    Assateague Island National Seashore, 136–38
    Assateague State Park, 143–45
Big Pool, Fort Frederick State Park, 42–44
Big Run Road, Savage River State Forest, 84–86
Big Run State Park, 10–12
Big Slackwater, C&O Canal, 27
Big Woods, C&O Canal, 27
Biking, 7–8
    Assateague Island National Seashore, 134–36
    C&O Canal, 23–26, 27–29
    Green Ridge State Forest, 57–59
    Patapsco Valley State Park, 120–22, 123–25
Billy Goat Trail, C&O Canal, 24
Birding
    Assateague Island National Seashore, 134–36
    Elk Neck State Park, 108–10
    Martinak State Park, 149–51
    Patuxent River Park, 126–28
    Pocomoke River State Park, 152–54
    Susquehanna State Park, 129–31
    Tuckahoe State Park, 164–66
Blackwater Canoe Trail, Pocomoke River State Park, 155–57
Blue Ridge Summit Overlook, 17
Blue Trail, Elk Neck State Park, 108–10
Boating and canoeing
    Assateague Island National Seashore
        backcountry sites, 139–42
        Bayside Campground, 134–36
        Oceanside Campground, 136–38
    Big Run State Park, 10–12
    Brunswick Family Campground, 13–15
    C&O Canal
        drive-in sites, 19–22
        Horseshoe Bend to Cacapon Junction, 27–29
        Swain's Lock to Killiansburg Cave, 23–26
    Cunningham Falls State Park, 33–35
    Deep Creek Lake State Park, 39–41
    Elk Neck State Park, 108–10
    Fort Frederick State Park, 42–44
    Green Ridge State Forest, 60–62
    Hart Miller Island, 114–16
    Janes Island State Park, 146–48
    Louise F. Cosca Regional Park, 102–4
    Maple Tree Camp, 66–68
    New Germany State Park, 69–71
    Patapsco Valley State Park, 123–25

Boating and canoeing (*continued*)
  Patuxent River Park, 126–28
  Pocomoke River State Park, 152–54, 155–57
  Point Lookout State Park, 158–60
  Savage River State Forest, 81–83
  Tuckahoe State Park, 164–66
  Youghiogheny River, 97–99
Bob's Hill, Cunningham Falls State Park, 33–35
Bogs, Cedarville, 105–7
Boonsboro
  Greenbrier State Park, 63–65
  South Mountain State Park, 87–90, 91–93
Brandywine, Cedarville State Forest, 105–7
Brown Trail, Cedarville State Forest, 105–7
Brunswick Family Campground, 13–15
Brunswick Railroad Museum, 66
Burkittsville, Maple Tree Camp, 66–68
Buzzard's Rock Trail, Patapsco Valley State Park, 120–22

C&O Canal, 23–26
  drive-in sites, 19–22
  Fort Frederick State Park, 42–44
  hiker/biker sites
    Horseshoe Bend to Cacapon Junction, 27–29
    Indigo Neck to Evitts Creek, 30–32
    Swain's Lock to Killiansburg Cave, 23–26
C&O Canal National Historic Park Visitor Center, 13
Cabins, New Germany State Park, 69–71
Cacapon Junction, C&O Canal, 27–29
Calico Rocks, C&O Canal, 26
Camp David, Catoctin Mountain Park, 16–18
Campfire programs, Deep Creek Lake State Park, 40
Camping equipment, 171
Canoeing. *See* Boating and canoeing
Casselman River, Savage River State Forest, 81–83
Cat Rock, Cunningham Falls State Park, 33–35
Catoctin Iron Furnace, Cunningham Falls State Park, 36–38
Catoctin Mountain Park, 16–18
Catoctin Mountains, 33–35
Catoctin Trail, 45–47
Catoctin Wildlife Preserve and Zoo, 34–35
Caves
  Crystal Grottoes, 66
  Killiansburg, 23–26
Cedarville State Forest, 105–7
Central Maryland, 101–34
Charcoal Trail, Patapsco Valley State Park, 121–22
Chesapeake Bay
  Elk Neck State Park, 108–10
  Hart Miller Island, 114–16
  Janes Island State Park, 146–48
  Martinak State Park, 149–51
  Point Lookout State Park, 158–60
  Smallwood State Park, 161–63
Children's activities. *See* Family camping

Chimney Rock, Cunningham Falls State Park, 17, 33–35
Chincoteague, Virginia, 134–36
Chisel Branch, C&O Canal, 24
Choptank River
  Martinak State Park, 149–51
  Tuckahoe State Park, 164–66
Civil War Correspondent's Memorial, 67
Civil War sites. *See* Military sites
Clarksburg, Little Bennett Regional Park, 117–19
Clinton Regional Park (now Louise F. Cosca Regional Park), 102–4
Concerts, Janes Island State Park, 146–48
Conowingo Dam, 129–31
Conoy, Lake, Point Lookout State Park, 158–60
Coordinates, 2–3. *See also specific campgrounds*
Corkers Creek, Pocomoke River State Park, 155–57
Cosca, Louise F., Regional Park, 102–4
Crabbing, Assateague Island National Seashore, 136–38
Crampton Gap, South Mountain State Park, 88–90
Cranesville Swamp, Garrett State Forest, 51–53
Crisfield, Janes Island State Park, 146–48
Croom Airfield, Patuxent River Park, 126–28
Crystal Grottoes Caverns, 66
Cumberland, 32
Cunningham Falls State Park, 16
  Houck Area, 33–35
  Manor Area, 36–38
Cypress Swamp, 152–54

Dahlgren, South Mountain State Park, 91–93
Darlington, Susquehanna State Park, 129–31
Daugherty Creek, Janes Island State Park, 147–48
Deep Creek Lake State Park, Meadow Mountain Campground, 39–41
Deer Park, Potomac State Forest
  Laurel Run and Wallman Areas, 75–77
  Lostland Run Area and Back Country, 72–74
Deer Spring Branch, Cunningham Falls State Park, 34–35
Denton, Martinak State Park, 149–51
Devil's Alley, C&O Canal, 30–32
Devil's Backbone County Park, 67
Devil's Racecourse, South Mountain State Park, 88–90
Discover Center, Deep Creek Lake State Park, 40
Douglass, Frederick, 164–66
Dunes, Assateague State Park, 143–45

Eastern Shore, 135–66
Ed Garvey, South Mountain State Park, 88–90
Edwards Ferry, C&O Canal, 24
Elk Lick Area, Savage River State Forest, 82–83
Elk Neck State Park, 108–10
Ellicott City, Patapsco Valley State Park
  Hilton Area, 120–22
  Hollofield Area, 123–25

Ensign Cowall, South Mountain State Park, 88–90
Equestrian trails. *See* Horseback riding
Equipment, camping, 171
Etiquette, camping, 7
Evitts Creek, C&O Canal, 30–32
Evitts Mountain, Rocky Gap State Park, 78–80

Facilities. *See specific campgrounds,* key information
Falls. *See* Waterfalls
Family camping
    Brunswick Family Campground, 13–15
    Cedarville State Forest, 105–7
    Cunningham Falls State Park, 33–35
    Elk Neck State Park, 108–10
    Janes Island State Park, 146–48
    Little Bennett Regional Park, 117–19
    Louise F. Cosca Regional Park, 102–4
    Patapsco Valley State Park
        Hilton Area, 120–22
        Hollofield Area, 123–25
    Point Lookout State Park, 158–60
    Smallwood State Park, 161–63
Farm museums, 129–31
Fifteen Mile Creek, C&O Canal, 19–22,
    30–32
Fire regulations. *See specific campgrounds,* key
    information
First-aid kit, 4
Fishing
    Big Run State Park, 10–12
    Brunswick Family Campground, 13–15
    Cedarville State Forest, 105–7
    Cunningham Falls State Park, 33–35, 36–38
    Deep Creek Lake State Park, 39–41
    Elk Neck State Park, 108–10
    Fort Frederick State Park, 42–44
    Gambrill State Park, 45–47
    Green Ridge State Forest, 57–59
    Greenbrier State Park, 63–65
    Hart Miller Island, 114–16
    Louise F. Cosca Regional Park, 102–4
    Martinak State Park, 149–51
    New Germany State Park, 69–71
    Patapsco Valley State Park, 120–22, 123–25
    Savage River State Forest, 81–83
    Smallwood State Park, 161–63
    Susquehanna State Park, 129–31
    Swallow Falls State Park, 94–96
    Youghiogheny River, 97–99
Flintstone
    Green Ridge State Forest, 60–62
        North of I-68, 54–56
        West of Green Ridge, 57–59
    Rocky Gap State Park, 78–80
Fort Frederick, C&O Canal, 28
Fort Frederick State Park, 42–44
Frederick, Gambrill State Park, 45–47
Friendsville, Youghiogheny River Lake, 97–99

Gambrill State Park, Rock Run Area, 45–47
Gapland, Maple Tree Camp, 66–68
Garrett State Forest
    Piney Mountain Area and Back Country, 51–53
    Snaggy Mountain Area, 48–50
Geography, 1
Georgetown Visitor's Center, C&O Canal, 19
Global coordinates, 2–3. *See also specific campgrounds*
Golf, Rocky Gap State Park, 78–80
Gorges, Mather, 24
Grantsville
    Big Run State Park, 10–12
    New Germany State Park, 69–71
    Savage River State Forest, 81–83, 84–86
Great Falls, C&O Canal, 23–26
Green Ridge State Forest
    East of Green Ridge, 60–62
    North of I-68, 54–56
    West of Green Ridge, 57–59
Green Trail, Cedarville State Forest, 105–7
Greenbelt Park, 111–13
Greenbrier State Park, 63–65
Grist mill, Susquehanna State Park, 129–31
Grist Mill Trail, Patapsco Valley State Park, 121–22

Habeeb, Lake, 78–80
Hagerstown, C&O Canal, 19–22
Hancock, C&O Canal, 28
Harpers Ferry, West Virginia, 13, 66–68
Hart Miller Island, 114–16
Hawk's Reach Activity Center, Little Bennett
    Regional Park, 117–19
Hazards, 4–5
Heron Alley Trail, Point Lookout State Park, 158–60
Herrington Manor, 48–50, 94–96
High Knob, Gambrill State Park, 45–47
Hiking
    Assateague Island National Seashore, 136–38
    Big Run State Park, 10–12
    C&O Canal
        drive-in sites, 19–22
        Horseshoe Bend to Cacapon Junction, 27–29
        Swain's Lock to Killiansburg Cave, 23–26
    Catoctin Mountain Park, 16–18
    Cunningham Falls State Park, 33–35, 36–38
    Deep Creek Lake State Park, 39–41
    Elk Neck State Park, 108–10
    Fort Frederick State Park, 42–44
    Gambrill State Park, 45–47
    Garrett State Forest, 48–50
    Green Ridge State Forest, 57–59
    Greenbrier State Park, 63–65
    Hart Miller Island, 114–16
    Janes Island State Park, 146–48
    Maple Tree Camp, 66–68
    Martinak State Park, 149–51
    Patapsco Valley State Park, 120–22, 123–25
    Patuxent River Park, 126–28

Hiking (*continued*)
Pocomoke River State Park, 152–54
Point Lookout State Park, 158–60
Rocky Gap State Park, 78–80
South Mountain State Park, 87–90
Susquehanna State Park, 129–31
Swallow Falls State Park, 94–96
tips for, 7–8
Tuckahoe State Park, 164–66
Hilton Area, Patapsco Valley State Park, 120–22
Historic sites
Cunningham Falls State Park, 36–38
Fort Frederick State Park, 42–44
Janes Island State Park, 146–48
Maple Tree Camp, 66–68
Martinak State Park, 149–51
Point Lookout State Park, 158–60
Smallwood State Park, 161–63
South Mountain State Park, 91–93
Susquehanna State Park, 129–31
Tuckahoe State Park, 164–66
Hollofield Area, Patapsco Valley State Park, 123–25
Horseback riding
Green Ridge State Forest, 58–59, 60–62
Patapsco Valley State Park, 123–25
Patuxent River Park, 126–28
Horsepen Branch, C&O Canal, 24
Horses, wild
Assateague Island National Seashore, 134–36,
136–38
Assateague State Park, 143–45
Horseshoe Bend, C&O Canal, 27–29
Houck Area, Cunningham Falls State Park, 33–35
Huckleberry Hill, C&O Canal, 26
Hunting, Patapsco Valley State Park, 123–25
Hunting Creek Lake, 33–35
Hypothermia, 8

Indian Flats, C&O Canal, 24–25
Indigo Neck, C&O Canal, 30–32
Information resources, 5, 169
Insects, Assateague Island National Seashore,
136–38, 141
Iron furnace, Cunningham Falls State Park, 36–38
Irons Mountain, C&O Canal, 31–32

Janes Island State Park, 146–48
Jordan Junction, C&O Canal, 28
Jug Bay Natural Area, Patuxent River Park, 127–28

Kayaking. *See* Boating and canoeing
Keysers Ridge, Savage River State Forest, 85–86
Killiansburg Cave, C&O Canal, 23–26

Lake(s)
Conowingo Dam, 129–31
Conoy, 158–60
Deep Creek, 39–41

Greenbrier, 63–65
Habeeb, 78–80
Herrington Manor, 48–50
Hunting Creek, 33–35
Louise F. Cosca Regional Park, 102–4
New Germany, 69–71
Savage River Reservoir, 10–12, 81–83, 84–86
Tuckahoe State Park, 164–66
Youghiogheny River, 97–99
Laurel Run, Potomac State Forest, 75–77
Leopards Mill, C&O Canal, 28
License, fishing, 170
Licking Creek, C&O Canal, 28
Life of the Forest Trail, Assateague Island National
Seashore, 137
Lighthouse, Turkey Point, 108–10
Lighthouse Trail, Point Lookout State Park, 158–60
Little Annemessex River, Janes Island State Park,
147–48
Little Bennett Regional Park, 117–19
Little Hunting Creek, Cunningham Falls State Park,
36–38
Little Levels, Assateague Island National Seashore,
139–42
Little Orleans, C&O Canal, 30–32
Little Pool Mile, C&O Canal, 28
Little Tonoloway, C&O Canal, 28–29
Lostland Run Area and Back Country, Potomac
State Forest, 72–74
Louise F. Cosca Regional Park, 102–4

McCoy's Ferry, C&O Canal, 19–22, 28
McMahon's Mill, C&O Canal, 27
Manor Area, Cunningham Falls State Park, 36–38
Maple Tree Camp, 66–68
Maps, overview, 2
Marble Quarry, C&O Canal, 24–25
Marbury, Smallwood State Park, 161–63
Margraff Trails, Savage River State Forest, 85–86
Marlton, Patuxent River Park, 126–28
Martinak State Park, 149–51
Mather Gorge, C&O Canal, 24
Mattawoman Creek, Smallwood State Park, 161–63
Meadow Mountain Campground, Deep Creek Lake
State Park, 39–41
Milburn Landing Area, Pocomoke River State Park,
152–54
Military sites
Brunswick Family Campground, 13–15
C&O Canal, 19–22
Fort Frederick State Park, 42–44
Gambrill State Park, 45–47
Maple Tree Camp, 66–68
Point Lookout State Park, 158–60
South Mountain State Park, 91–93
Mill Run Campground, Youghiogheny River Lake,
97–99
Monocacy, C&O Canal, 24–25

Monroe Run Trail, 11
Mosquitoes, 5
  Assateague Island National Seashore, 136–38, 141
Muddy Creek Falls, 94–96
Museums
  farm, 129–31
  Patuxent River Park, 126–28
  railroad, 13–15
  railroad museums, 66

Nassawango Creek, 152–54
Native American sites
  Cedarville State Forest, 105–7
  Martinak State Park, 149–51
  Susquehanna State Park, 129–31
Nature centers and trails
  Deep Creek Lake State Park, 40
  Little Bennett Regional Park, 117–19
  Patapsco Valley State Park, 123–25
Negro Mountain, 85–86
New Germany State Park, 69–71
Noland's Ferry, C&O Canal, 24–25
North Branch, C&O Canal, 31–32
North East, Elk Neck State Park, 108–10
North Mountain, C&O Canal, 28

Oakland
  Garrett State Forest, 48–50
  Swallow Falls State Park, 94–96
Oceanside Campground, Assateague Island
    National Seashore, 136–38
Off-roading, Assateague Island National Seashore,
    136–38
Old Town Road, Green Ridge State Forest, 60–62
Ole Ranger Trail, Patapsco Valley State Park,
    123–25
Opequon Junction, C&O Canal, 27
Orchard Pond, Green Ridge State Forest, 60–62
Outflow, Youghiogheny River Lake, 97–99
Overlooks
  Blue Ridge Summit, 17
  Potomac, 72–74
Owens Creek Campground, Catoctin Mountain
    Park, 17

Parking. *See specific campgrounds,* key information
Patapsco Valley State Park
  Hilton Area, 120–22
  Hollofield Area, 123–25
Patuxent River Park, 126–28
Paw Paw, West Virginia, C&O Canal, 19–22
Paw Paw Tunnel, C&O Canal, 30–32
Peaceful Pond Trail, Patapsco Valley State Park,
    123–25
Pen Mar, South Mountain State Park, 91–93
Periwinkle Point Trail, Point Lookout State Park,
    158–60
Permits, 7

Pets. *See specific campgrounds,* key information
Pigman's Ferry, C&O Canal, 31–32
Pine Knob, South Mountain State Park, 88–90
Pine Lick Trail, Green Ridge State Forest, 54–56
Piney Mountain Area and Back Country, Garrett
    State Forest, 51–53
Pirate Island, Assateague Island National Seashore,
    141
Plant hazards, 5
Playgrounds
  Louise F. Cosca Regional Park, 102–4
  Patapsco Valley State Park, 123–25
  Smallwood State Park, 161–63
Pocomoke River State Park
  Milburn Landing Area, 152–54
  Shad Landing Area, 155–57
Pogo, South Mountain State Park, 91–93
Point Lookout State Park, 158–60
Point of Rocks, C&O Canal, 26
Poison ivy, 5
Polish Mountain, Green Ridge State Forest, 54,
    57–59
Ponies, wild
  Assateague Island National Seashore, 134–36,
    136–38
  Assateague State Park, 143–45
Pope Bay, Assateague Island National Seashore,
    139–42
Poplar Lick
  New Germany State Park, 69–71
  Savage River State Forest, 82–83
Potomac Forks, C&O Canal, 31–32
Potomac Overlook, 72–74
Potomac River
  Brunswick Family Campground, 13–15
  C&O Canal
    drive-in sites, 19–22
    Horseshoe Bend to Cacapon Junction, 27–29
    Indigo Neck to Evitts Creek, 30–32
    Swain's Lock to Killiansburg Cave, 23–26
  Fort Frederick State Park, 42–44
  Garrett State Forest, 48–50
  Maple Tree Camp, 66–68
  Point Lookout State Park, 158–60
Potomac State Forest
  Laurel Run and Wallman Areas, 75–77
  Lostland Run Area and Back Country, 72–74
Purslane Run, C&O Canal, 31–32

Queen Anne, Tuckahoe State Park, 164–66

Rafting, Youghiogheny River, 97–99
Railroad museums, 13–15, 66
Rails-To-Trails Conservancy, 42
Registration. *See specific campgrounds,*
    key information
Restrictions. *See specific campgrounds,* key information
Riding trails. *See* Horseback riding

River Ridge Trail, Patapsco Valley State Park, 123–25
Rock formations
  C&O Canal, 26
  Cunningham Falls State Park, 33–35
  Greenbrier State Park, 63–65
  Patapsco Valley State Park, 121–22
  South Mountain State Park, 91–93
Rock Run Area, Gambrill State Park, 45–47
Rock Run Historical Area, Susquehanna State Park, 129–31
Rock Run Mansion, 129–31
Rocky Gap State Park, 78–80
Rocky Point Marina, Hart-Miller Island, 114–16
Rocky Run, South Mountain State Park, 88–90
Roosevelt, Franklin D, Catoctin Mountain Park, 16–18
Round Top Cement Mill, C&O Canal, 28

Safety, 7–8
Sand dunes, Assateague State Park, 143–45
Sang Run, Garrett State Forest, 51–53
Santee Branch Trail, Patapsco Valley State Park, 121–22
Savage River Reservoir, 10–12
Savage River State Forest, 82–83
  Northeast of Savage River Reservoir, 81–83
  Reservoir and Big Run North, 84–86
Sawmill Branch Trail, Patapsco Valley State Park, 121–22
Scotland, Point Lookout State Park, 158–60
Seneca Creek State Park, 24
Shad Landing Area, Pocomoke River State Park, 155–57
Shangri-La (Franklin D. Roosevelt retreat), Catoctin Mountain Park, 16–18
Sharpsburg, C&O Canal, 27–29
Shelters
  Catoctin Mountain Park, 17
  South Mountain State Park, 87–90
Sideling Hill Creek
  C&O Canal, 30–32
  Green Ridge State Forest, 60–62
Sideling Hill Visitor Center, 20
Sinepuxent Bay
  Assateague Island National Seashore, 133–34
  Assateague State Park, 143–45
Smallwood State Park, 161–63
Smith, John, 129, 146
Snaggy Mountain Area, Garrett State Forest, 48–50
Snakes, 4
Snow Hill, Pocomoke River State Park
  Milburn Landing Area, 152–54
  Shad Landing Area, 155–57
Sorrel Ridge Mile, C&O Canal, 30–32
South Mountain
  Gambrill State Park, 45–47
  Maple Tree Camp, 66–68

South Mountain State Park/Appalachian Trail
  backpackers' campgrounds, 91–93
  trail shelters, 87–90
South Ocean Beach, Assateague Island National Seashore, 136–38
Southern Maryland, 135–66
Sports
  Louise F. Cosca Regional Park, 102–4
  Patuxent River Park, 126–28
Spring Gap, C&O Canal, 19–22, 31–32
State Line, Assateague Island National Seashore, 139–42
Stay limits. See specific campgrounds, key information
Steppingstone Museum, 129–31
Stream crossing, 8
Summer Park Pal program, Janes Island State Park, 146–48
Susquehanna State Park, 129–31
Swain's Lock, C&O Canal, 23–26
Swallow Falls State Park, 48–50, 94–96
Swamps
  Cranesville, 51–53
  Cypress, 152–54
  Zekiah, 105–7
Swanton, Deep Creek Lake State Park, 39–41
Sweden Point Marina, Smallwood State Park, 161–63
Swimming
  Assateague Island National Seashore, 136–38, 139–42
  C&O Canal, 19–22
  Deep Creek Lake State Park, 39–41
  Elk Neck State Park, 108–10
  Fort Frederick State Park, 42–44
  Hart Miller Island, 114–16
  Maple Tree Camp, 66–68
  New Germany State Park, 69–71
  Point Lookout State Park, 158–60
Sycamore Landing, C&O Canal, 24

Tangier Sound, 146–48
Tanner's Creek, Point Lookout State Park, 158–60
Tennis, Louise F. Cosca Regional Park, 102–4
Thurmont
  Catoctin Mountain Park, 16–18
  Cunningham Falls State Park, 33–35, 36–38
Thurmont Vista, 17
Ticks, 4–5
Tingles Narrows, Assateague Island National Seashore, 141
Tolliver Falls, 94–96
Toms Cove, Virginia, 136–38
Town Creek, C&O Canal, 31–32
Town Hill, Green Ridge State Forest, 54, 57–59
Towpath, C&O. See C&O Canal
Trail shelters
  Appalachian Trail, 87–90
  Catoctin Mountain Park, 17

Trains, miniature, 102–4
Treehouses, Maple Tree Camp, 66–68
Tub Run, Youghiogheny River Lake, 97–99
Tuckahoe State Park, 164–66
Tunnel Hill Trail, C&O Canal, 30–32
Tunnels, C&O Canal, 30–32
Turkey Point Lighthouse, 108–10
Turtle Run, C&O Canal, 24–25

Underground Railroad, Tuckahoe State Park,
    164–66
UTM coordinates, 2–3

Wallman Area, Potomac State Forest, 75–77
Ward Creek, Janes Island State Park, 147–48
Warrior Mountain, 22, 31–32, 58
Washington, D. C.
    Catoctin Mountain Park, 16–18
    Greenbelt Park, 111–13
    Little Bennett Regional Park, 117–19
    Smallwood State Park, 161–63
Washington Monument State Park, 63
Waterfalls
    C&O Canal, 23–26
    Cunningham, 33–35
    Cunningham Falls State Park, 36–38
    Muddy Creek, 94–96
    Swallow, 48–50
    Swallow Falls State Park, 94–96
    Tolliver, 94–96

Watts Creek, Martinak State Park, 149–51
Western Maryland, 9–99
Western Maryland Rail Trail, 42
Weverton, South Mountain State Park, 91–93
White Rock, C&O Canal, 28
White Sulphur Pond, Green Ridge State Forest,
    58–59
White's Ferry, C&O Canal, 24–25
Whitewater sports, Youghiogheny River, 97–99
Wicomico River, Cedarville State Forest, 105–7
Wild horses, Assateague Island National Seashore,
    134–36, 137–38
Wildflowers, Cedarville State Forest, 105–7
Wildlife
    Assateague State Park, 144–46
    Cedarville State Forest, 105–7
    Janes Island State Park, 147–48
    Pocomoke River State Park, 153–55
    Tuckahoe State Park, 165–66
William Houck Area, Cunningham Falls State Park,
    33–35
Williamsport, C&O Canal, 27–28
Wolf Rock, Cunningham Falls State Park, 17, 33–35

Youghiogheny River, 94–96
Youghiogheny River Lake, Mill Run Campground,
    97–99

Zekiah Swamp, Cedarville State Forest, 105–7
Zoos, Cunningham Falls State Park, 34–35

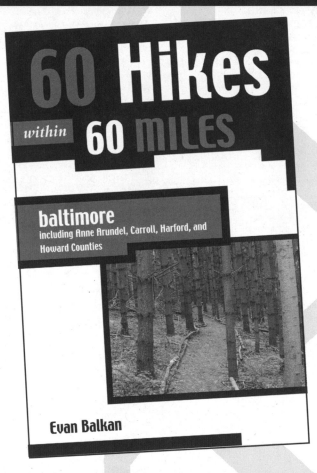

DEAR CUSTOMERS AND FRIENDS,

SUPPORTING YOUR INTEREST IN OUTDOOR ADVENTURE, travel, and an active lifestyle is central to our operations, from the authors we choose to the locations we detail to the way we design our books. Menasha Ridge Press was incorporated in 1982 by a group of veteran outdoorsmen and professional outfitters. For 25 years now, we've specialized in creating books that benefit the outdoors enthusiast.

Almost immediately, Menasha Ridge Press earned a reputation for revolutionizing outdoors- and travel-guidebook publishing. For such activities as canoeing, kayaking, hiking, backpacking, and mountain biking, we established new standards of quality that transformed the whole genre, resulting in outdoor-recreation guides of great sophistication and solid content. Menasha Ridge continues to be outdoor publishing's greatest innovator.

The folks at Menasha Ridge Press are as at home on a white-water river or mountain trail as they are editing a manuscript. The books we build for you are the best they can be, because we're responding to your needs. Plus, we use and depend on them ourselves.

We look forward to seeing you on the river or the trail. If you'd like to contact us directly, join in at www.trekalong.com or visit us at www.menasharidge.com. We thank you for your interest in our books and the natural world around us all.

SAFE TRAVELS,

BOB SEHLINGER
PUBLISHER